The
Family
Pharmacist

An A–Z Guide to
Children's Illnesses and
Medications

The
Family
Pharmacist

An A–Z Guide to
Children's Illnesses and
Medications

LISA M. CHAVIS, R.PH.

A Perigee Book

THE BERKLEY PUBLISHING GROUP
Published by the Penguin Group
Penguin Group (USA) Inc.
375 Hudson Street, New York, New York 10014, USA
Penguin Group (Canada), 10 Alcorn Avenue, Toronto, Ontario M4V 3B2, Canada
(a division of Pearson Penguin Canada Inc.)
Penguin Books Ltd., 80 Strand, London WC2R 0RL, England
Penguin Group Ireland, 25 St. Stephen's Green, Dublin 2, Ireland (a division of Penguin Books Ltd.)
Penguin Group (Australia), 250 Camberwell Road, Camberwell, Victoria 3124, Australia
(a division of Pearson Australia Group Pty. Ltd.)
Penguin Books India Pvt. Ltd., 11 Community Centre, Panchsheel Park, New Delhi—110 017, India
Penguin Group (NZ), Cnr. Airborne and Rosedale Roads, Albany, Auckland 1310, New Zealand
(a division of Pearson New Zealand Ltd.)
Penguin Books (South Africa) (Pty.) Ltd., 24 Sturdee Avenue, Rosebank, Johannesburg 2196, South Africa

Penguin Books Ltd., Registered Offices: 80 Strand, London WC2R 0RL, England

This book is an original publication of The Berkley Publishing Group.

While the author has made every effort to provide accurate telephone numbers and Internet addresses at the time of publication, neither the publisher nor the author assumes any responsibility for errors, or for changes that occur after publication.

First edition: March 2005

Library of Congress Cataloging-in-Publication Data

Chavis, Lisa M.
    The family pharmacist : an A-Z guide to children's illnesses and medications / Lisa Chavis.
        p.   cm.
    ISBN 0-399-53075-4
        1. Children—Health and hygiene—Encyclopedias.   2. Children—Diseases—Encyclopedias.
    3. Pediatrics—Formulae, receipts, prescriptions—Encyclopedias.   4. Drugs, Nonprescription—
    Encyclopedias.   I. Title.

    RJ61.C533 2005
    618.92'003—dc22

                                                                          2004057680

PRINTED IN THE UNITED STATES OF AMERICA

10   9   8   7   6   5   4   3   2   1

Dedication

For each lost paper found, for every misplaced reference book located, for every random thought focused, and for all those computer files recovered, a special THANK YOU to Cheryl MacDonald. My best friend and organizer extraordinaire!

Acknowledgments

Having the opportunity to have a book published is an amazing gift. Thank you again and again to my editor, Sheila Curry Oakes, editorial assistant Adrienne Schultz, and my agent, Rita Rosenkranz, for seeing promise in my work and ensuring that it found a place on the bookshelf.

Families, like children, come in many different forms. *The Family Pharmacist* acknowledges the wonderful job parents and caregivers of all types are doing to ensure the health and safety of one of our most precious resources.

Contents

Part One
Hot Topics

Part Two
Fingertip Advisors:
Fast Guidance for Childhood Ailments

Appendices

Introduction

Today many parents come to the pharmacy counter with questions about their children's health and their children's medications. Questions are asked about head lice, chicken pox, poison ivy, and upset tummies—all before noon. Some days I feel as though there must be several epidemics going on in the daycare set! This book was written with these parents and caregivers in mind.

"Hot Topics" covers some of the more newsworthy health issues affecting children today. From how to prepare your family for a bioterrorism attack to what you can do as a parent to decrease the epidemic of antibiotic resistance, these topics provide relevant and timely information for your child's health.

"Fingertip Advisors" provide quick, concise, and easily accessible health information in an easy-to-understand manner. When your child is sick, you don't have time to search for information. Now you don't have to.

The over-the-counter medicine aisles can be a minefield for parents, with choices ranging from syrups to elixirs, suspensions, reditabs, chewables, tablets, creams, ointments, and sprays, and all with age-specific dosages and dosage forms. Parents must keep in mind that children aren't simply small adults, but have their own medication needs. Adult medicines can be harmful to young bodies, so proper dosing is important.

Newspapers and the Internet are rife with information about the latest medical news on children's conditions, like ADHD. What is the latest information? What about side effects of medicines? What is safe for your child? Parents express concern over the safety of vaccinations, as well as the safety of insect repellants and sunscreens. This book will answer your questions and ease your concerns.

While children certainly don't come with instruction books, this book is meant to be a parent-friendly instruction book for the world of children's health and children's medicine.

Best of health and best of life to your family!

—Lisa M. Chavis, R.Ph., AKA "The Drug Lady"

Who is the "Drug Lady"?

The "Drug Lady" name came from a dear customer who always came into the pharmacy looking for his "Drug Lady" to answer his questions about medicines. He said that his doctor didn't have the time and the books he read didn't explain things in terms he could understand.

Your "Drug Lady" is a registered community pharmacist with a background in over-the-counter medications, women's and children's health, and drug information. I answer questions daily from parents just like you who are concerned about making the best possible decisions for their children's health.

It is important to me that your family is healthy. With this in mind, please remember the information in this book should in no way replace the advice of your child's own doctor. He/she is more familiar with your child's specific medical history and can make the best recommendations based on that information.

The
Family
Pharmacist

An A–Z Guide to
Children's Illnesses and
Medications

PART ONE

Hot Topics

1

ADHD

ADHD is the most common of childhood chronic conditions, and also raises the most controversy. There are two distinct camps in the ADHD battle: those who feel medication is the answer and those who do not. Increased public awareness of this condition and a decrease in tolerance of ADHD symptoms by society as a whole has led to a dramatic increase in the number of diagnoses and medications being prescribed for children. Some parents are concerned that their children are being overdiagnosed and overtreated. In this section, you'll be presented with the very valid points from both sides of the discussion. Once you have read these pages, you'll have the information at hand for making the best decision for your family situation.

The Definition of ADHD

Attention Deficit Hyperactivity Disorder (ADHD) is the most common psychiatric disorder affecting children and adolescents. There are three types of ADHD:

1. **Inattentive only disorder.** This was formerly called ADD (Attention Defecit Disorder). ADD was renamed in 1994 and placed un-

der the more umbrella term ADHD. With this type of disorder, the child has six or more symptoms of "inattention," as listed below.

2. Hyperactive/impulsive disorder. With this type of disorder, the child has six or more symptoms of "hyperactivity-impulsivity," as listed below.

3. Combined inattentive/hyperactive/impulsive disorder. With this disorder, the child has six or more symptoms of inattention and six or more symptoms of hyperactivity-impulsivity.

It is estimated that three to 20 percent of children are diagnosed with these conditions. That breaks down to approximately one child with ADHD in every school classroom in the United States.

INATTENTION SYMPTOMS:

- Often failing to pay attention to details or making careless mistakes in schoolwork, work, or other activities.
- Often having difficulty sustaining attention in tasks or play.
- Often not listening when spoken to directly.
- Often not following through on instructions and failing to finish a project.
- Often having difficulty organizing tasks and activities.
- Often avoiding, disliking, or being reluctant to engage in tasks that require sustained mental effort.
- Often losing things necessary for tasks or activities.
- Often being distracted by extraneous stimuli.
- Often being forgetful in daily activities.

HYPERACTIVITY-IMPULSIVITY SYMPTOMS:

Hyperactivity Symptoms:

- Often fidgeting with hands or feet, or squirming in a seat.
- Often inappropriately leaving a seat in the classroom or in other situations.
- Often running or climbing excessively in situations in which it is inappropriate.
- Often having difficulty playing or engaging in leisure activities quietly.
- Often being "on the go" or acting as if "driven by a motor."
- Often talking excessively.

IMPULSIVITY SYMPTOMS:

- Often blurting out answers before questions have been completed.
- Often having difficulty awaiting a turn.
- Often interrupting or intruding on others.

The Causes of ADHD

Unfortunately, there is no one particular area to pinpoint as the cause for ADHD. However, there are many theories. What we do know is ADHD seems to run in families. Twin and family studies show the strong familial tie, possibly traced to a specific gene for ADHD. If a parent carries that specific gene, it may be passed to their child or children.

Abnormal levels of certain brain chemicals or neurotransmitters have also been linked to ADHD. Studies have shown that children with ADHD have less brain electrical activity and show less reaction to stimulation in one or more regions of the brain.

Other possible causes of ADHD are low birth weight, brain injury at birth, fetal alcohol syndrome, heavy metal poisoning, extreme reaction to particular foods, and exposure of the unborn baby to nicotine.

The Risk Factors of ADHD

Boys are two to three times as likely as girls to be diagnosed with ADHD. However, girls are closing the gap in the area of inattentive-based ADHD. Children with ADHD are more likely to experience social dysfunction, academic problems, and difficulty at home. Because ADHD children are often extremely bright, this disorder does not appear to affect intelligence. However, studies suggest that 90 percent of ADHD-diagnosed children are underachievers and that 50 percent are held back in school at least one year. Reading difficulties persist in 20 percent of cases and serious handwriting problems can be found in 60 percent of cases. Studies conducted with parents of ADHD children show persistence of ADHD from childhood to adolescence in 60 to 80 percent of cases.

Up to 66 percent of children with ADHD are diagnosed with a second disorder as well, while nearly 33 percent of children with ADHD have more than two conditions. You might hear this referred to as comorbidity. Comorbid disorders commonly seen with ADHD are oppositional defiant disorder (ODD), conduct disorder, dyslexia, anxiety, depression, bipolar disorder, Tourette's syndrome, or learning disabilities.

In a community sample of six to 12 year olds with ADHD, oppositional defiant or conduct disorder appeared 25 to 35 percent of the time, anxiety disorders 26 percent, dyslexia 20 percent, mood disorders 18 percent, and learning disabilities 12 percent.

Age also factors in how the child displays behavioral problems. A younger onset age of ADHD is more likely to be associated with conduct disorders. As a child gets older, the symptoms manifest as emotional problems.

The Symptoms and Diagnosis of ADHD

There are three basic symptoms of ADHD: inattentiveness, hyperactivity, and impulsiveness not appropriate for a child of that age. The signs of inattention include not finishing assigned tasks, not paying attention or listening, not following directions, and being unable to focus to avoid making careless mistakes or becoming distracted. The hyperactivity aspect of ADHD can appear as constant interruptions while others are speaking, fidgeting, bursting into games or other activities already in progress without being invited, or talking excessively. Impulsiveness in an ADHD child is evidenced by the appearance of a lack of fear of pain or other consequences that may cause harm.

Many of these behaviors sound like the normal activities of every child from time to time. It is only when these symptoms appear before the age of seven and persist for over six months in a way that causes impairment to the child that ADHD might be addressed as the culprit.

Information used to diagnose the condition may include an interview with the child with a complete medical history, as well as asking a parent about the social, emotional, educational, and behavioral history of the child. A physical exam may be given to rule out any organic medical problems. A checklist for behaviors that may be linked to ADHD is given to parents and teachers to evaluate the child's symptoms.

THE PARENT'S PERSPECTIVE

Parenting a child with ADHD can be a daunting experience. The household may seem to be in a state of upheaval due to the constant needs of an ADHD child. Relationships between parents can become strained as they cope with different strategies for discipline and rewards for positive behavior.

Because many parents of ADHD children have undiagnosed or untreated ADHD themselves, it can be difficult for them to focus and organize tasks, like giving medications regularly or setting up daily schedules to follow. In addition, due to the strong genetic factor of ADHD, there is likely to be another child in the same household with the same condition. For siblings who do not have ADHD, the time and attention parents spend with the more disruptive child takes away from the time enjoyed by the entire family together.

As a parent, you realize this disorder can last many years. Prior thinking on ADHD was that it would be outgrown by the time the child reached young adulthood. However, recent studies now show ADHD follows a child into adolescence in 60 to 80 percent of children and into adulthood in up to 66 percent of children. There must be long-term commitment for treatment and extra assistance from everyone involved, including the child, caregivers, and the family unit.

It often helps if the family as a whole embraces the child's condition as a disability, not simply a willful conduct problem. The family may require training and classes to learn ways to deal with the child and his disability. With an ADHD child, there are many bright moments, and with the proper tools, the family unit can function together as one.

The Identification of ADHD

Regrettably, there is no blood test or exact method to determine whether a child has ADHD. The socially inappropriate symptoms must be used as a subjective determination of whether the child has the condition or not. Over the past few years, specific standards for ADHD diagnosis have been developed by organizations like The American Psychiatric Association (1994) and the American Academy of Pediatrics (2000). These standards have made it easier for physicians and clinicians to make a more accurate assessment of a child's behavior to determine if it is "just a phase" or ADHD.

DSM-IV STANDARDS

The Diagnostic and Statistical Manual of Mental Disorders, Fourth Edition is a manual published by the American Psychiatric Association that sets criteria for the diagnosis of neurobiologic and other psychiatric disorders, such as ADHD. The DSM-IV is the standard by which most referrals are made. The child's ADHD symptoms must be severe enough to cause improper social adaptation, be improper for his particular age level of development, and not be caused by another underlying condition. Impairment due to ADHD symptoms must be present in at least two different settings (for example, at home, in school, or at daycare).

Proper diagnosis requires documented problems of inattentiveness, restlessness, and impulsiveness from primary (parents) and secondary (teachers, coaches, daycare) caregivers. Because many of these behaviors are common in children, the child's problems must be abnormal for their age bracket and cause impairment in some aspect of daily life.

AAP CLINICAL PRACTICE GUIDELINES

In 2001, a more complete set of outcomes and guidelines for ADHD diagnosis and treatment was developed by the American Academy of Pediatrics (AAP).

The guidelines emphasize:

1. Consideration of ADHD as a chronic condition.

2. The use of symptom guidelines for diagnosis.

3. The use of medications and behavior therapy.

4. The close monitoring of treatment outcomes and failures.

Of particular debate in the ADHD battle is the third recommendation that a child be first prescribed a medication and/or appropriate behavioral therapy. This puts medication as the first choice for ADHD treatment. In part, the recommendation requires that the child's doctor should advise the use of a medication and/or behavior therapy, as appropriate, to improve symptoms and outcomes in children with ADHD.

AAP guidelines state physicians should begin with a low dose of medication and slowly increase it because there is a great deal of individual variability in how patients respond to the dose. Also, the first dose may improve a child's symptoms, but may not be the best dose to improve their functions. Physicians may use higher doses to achieve better responses, then reduce the dose when a higher dose produces side effects or no further improvement. If one medicine does not work at the highest feasible dose, the doctor may recommend another, until the core symptoms disappear.

TWO SIDES, ONE PROBLEM. ARE WE OVERMEDICATING OUR CHILDREN?

The use of prescription drugs is growing faster among children than it is among senior citizens and baby boomers, according to a survey by Medco Health Solutions, a Franklin Lakes, N.J.-based pharmacy benefits manager. Children are also spending 34 percent more time on medication than they did six years ago. Expenditures on medicines used to treat ADHD increased 122 percent over the past four years. In 2000, there was nearly a three-fold increase in the use of stimulant drugs among two to four year olds. This news is alarming for those who fear our children are being overmedicated.

There are two distinct camps in the battle against ADHD: those who prefer medicine to control the child's behavior and those who are opposed to medicating a child in any way. Public concerns have been made over the increased prevalence of ADHD diagnosis (and subsequent prescribing of medicines) for common childhood behavior problems in those as young as two years old.

The Long-term Effects of ADHD

Unfortunately, studies show that many cases of ADHD are not simply a childhood phase to be outgrown. More than half of children diagnosed with ADHD have other conditions to be dealt with, including conduct disorders, anxiety disorders, and depression. Manic depression (or bipolar disorder) also affects up to 25 percent of children with an ADHD diagnosis.

ADULT ADHD

Anywhere from ten to 60 percent of ADHD cases in childhood continue into adulthood, often with devastating effects on one's ability to hold a job, concentrate, or follow through with motivation. Adults tend to be less obviously hyperactive than young children, whose condition is clearly seen as running, talking, or playing out of turn. Adult variations of these symptoms include feeling uncomfortable sitting through meetings, being unwilling to wait in line, and speeding.

Parents concerned that they may have ADHD should talk to their own physician about symptoms including lack of focus, disorganization, restlessness, difficulty finishing projects, and/or losing things. An adult with ADHD may have difficulties at work, at home, and in their personal relationships. Adults diagnosed with ADHD must have had their first symptoms prior to age seven and these symptoms must have continued to cause impairment on a regular basis since then.

Medication Side Effects and Concerns

For the past 60 years, medication choices for treating ADHD have consisted of the short-acting brain stimulant variety (like Dexedrine or methylphenidate). Amphetamines used in the adult world as "diet drugs" or "speed" are commonly prescribed for children to curb the inappropriate social behaviors of ADHD. The AAP states that stimulants are generally considered safe medications, with few contraindications to their use. However, these medicines are listed as controlled substances due to their high potential for abuse by adults.

With the continued use of stimulant medications, side effects such as tic disorders can appear. Side effects occur early in treatment and tend to be mild and short-lived. The most common side effects are decreased appetite, stomachache or headache, delayed sleep onset, jitteriness, or social withdrawal. Appetite suppression and weight loss are common side effects of stimulant medication. Most of these symptoms can be successfully managed through adjustments in the dosage or schedule of medication. Approximately 15 to 30 percent of children experience motor tics, most of which are temporary, while on stimulant medications. Rarely, with high doses, some children experience psychotic reactions, mood disturbances, or hallucinations.

The ADHD Medication Arsenal

NONSTIMULANTS

Strattera (atomoxepine)

Newest on the market and offering promise because it is not a controlled substance or a mental stimulant, Strattera is changing the direction of ADHD treatment. This drug is the first nonstimulant medication approved for treating ADHD in children over the age of six, adolescents, and adults. The drug class is a selective norepinephrine reuptake inhibitor. In plain English, this drug changes the chemical balance in the brain to one more favorable for those diagnosed with ADHD.

It is usually taken once or twice daily: either in the morning or as a morning and late afternoon/evening combination. This is a plus for children who refuse to take medication during school hours. The most common side effects are upset stomach, decreased appetite, nausea/vomiting, dizziness, tiredness, or mood swings. Strattera can increase blood pressure and heart rate, and should be avoided in those with heart conditions, narrow angle glaucoma, or high blood pressure. It may also cause dizziness and fainting in children with low blood pressure. Other medicines, like the SSRI antidepressants Paxil (paroxitine) and Prozac (fluoxitine), can interact with Strattera and if used in combination with Strattera, should be discussed with the child's doctor.

A Drug Lady Reminder

Often we forget to mention over-the-counter medicines to the doctor when asked what other medications the child is taking. Before filling a prescription, it is very important to discuss with the doctor and pharmacist any and all medicines your child takes, even if only for an occasional sniffle, as some do have harmful interactions with each other.

ANTIDEPRESSANTS

Norpramine (desipramine) and Tofranil (imipramine)

Studies have shown that the tricyclic antidepressants, like desipramine or imipramine, can be used to treat ADHD symptoms effectively. In fact, four trials comparing tricyclic antidepressants with the stimulant Ritalin (methylphenidate) indicated either no differences in response or slightly better results with stimulant use.

Common side effects of tricyclic antidepressants include nervousness, sleep disorders, tiredness, and mild stomach upset. These typically go away during treatment. Less common side effects are constipation, convulsions, anxiety, and emotional instability. It is especially important to use extreme caution if combining these medicines with Ritalin. Ritalin can increase the levels of desipramine and imipramine in the child's blood and cause life-threatening side effects.

ANTIHYPERTENSIVES

Catapres (clonidine)

Limited studies of clonidine show it is better than a placebo (sugar pills), but less effective than stimulants in the treatment of ADHD symptoms. Its use has been mainly in children with ADHD and coexisting conditions, especially sleep disturbances. Side effects include dry mouth, drowsiness, dizziness, constipation, and sedation. With children in particular, it is extremely important that this medicine not be stopped abruptly without checking with the doctor. When suddenly stopped, side effects that may occur include nervousness, agitation, headaches, tremors, and a rapid increase in blood pressure. For children with an illness that causes vomiting, thus preventing them from keeping the medicine down, this rapid increase in blood pressure can be especially serious.

TYPES OF STIMULANTS

Short Acting—

Fast Onset of Action

Ritalin (methylphenidate)

Focalin (methylphenidate)

Adderal (mixed amphetamine salts)

Dextrostat (dextroamphetamine)

Dexedrine (dextroamphetamine)

Slower to Act—

Longer Duration in the System

Cylert (pemoline)

Metadate ER (methylphenidate)

Dexedrine Spansules (dextroamphetamine)

Fast Onset of Action—

Longer Duration in the System

Adderal XR (mixed amphetamine salts)

Metadate CD (methylphenidate)

Ritalin-LA (methylphenidate)

Concerta (methylphenidate)

STIMULANTS

Stimulant medications, despite the controversy, appear to be a safe and effective way of treating properly diagnosed ADHD children. In fact, nearly 80 percent of children treated with stimulants will respond favorably. Children taking these medications show improvement in areas of increased attention span, increased focus, ignoring distractions, and controlling inappropriate behaviors. There are several types of stimulants. The longer-acting varieties are preferred by school-aged children to avoid having to take a dose at school.

Side effects that may occur while taking stimulant medicine include decreased appetite (more severe in children), stomach upset, difficulty falling asleep, headache, nervousness, or dizziness. Less common side effects that should be discussed with the child's doctor include fever, joint pain, weight loss, irregular heartbeat, chest pain, vision changes or blurred vision, seizures, involuntary muscle movements, or changes in mood or personality. An allergic reaction to this medicine is unlikely, but seek immediate medical attention if it occurs. Symptoms of an allergic reaction include rash, itching, swelling, dizziness, or trouble breathing. If you notice these or any other unusual side effects, contact your child's doctor, nurse, or pharmacist.

The doctor may raise or lower your child's dose if he is also taking tricyclic antidepressants (for example, amitriptyline or nortriptyline), blood pressure medicine (for example, beta-blockers), other stimulant medications, guanethidine, meperidine, or urinary alkalinizers. Certain foods and drugs can affect the amount of acid in your child's stomach/intestine and may increase or decrease (depending on the drug) the absorption of this medicine. Tell your child's doctor if he is taking any of these products: fruit juices, ascorbic acid (vitamin C), sodium bicarbonate, ammonium chloride, sodium acid phosphate, anti-ulcer medicine (for example, H2 blockers, such as famotidine and ranitidine, or proton pump inhibitors [PPIs], such as omeprazole and lansoprazole), antacids, methenamine, and acetazolamide.

Children, adolescents, or adults should not use these medicines if they have heart disease or a blood vessel–related disease (for example, arteriosclerosis, cardiovascular disease), severe high blood pressure, overactive thyroid (hyperthyroidism), eye problems (for example, glaucoma), emotional instability, or a history of drug abuse. Inform your child's doctor of any other medical conditions such as other mental/mood problems (for example, psychological disorders), growth problems, high blood pressure, uncontrolled muscle movements (for example, tics, Tourette's syndrome), or allergies.

IS THE "ONE-SIZE FITS ALL" APPROACH THE BEST?

Since 1990, Ritalin (methylphenidate) use has risen 250 percent, according to the *Journal of the American Medical Association*. More than ten million prescriptions were written for Ritalin in 1996 and the trend is continuing upward.

Some experts believe that up to 90 percent of behavior problems are misdiagnosed as ADHD when the problem behavior may have an entirely different cause. Prescribing Ritalin as a first step in curbing inappropriate behavior may in fact be masking symptoms of another problem.

ADHD children are taught repeatedly to control their behavior and set limits with what is socially acceptable. If the child is suffering from depression or posttraumatic stress syndrome, the therapy is just the opposite. The child is encouraged to speak out and express their feelings. The treatments are vastly different, but the original symptoms are strikingly similar. The child may appear unfocused, inattentive, disruptive, or defiant.

The need for a quick solution for a child's disruptive behavior may overpower reasons to seek out deeper causes for the child's behavior. Childhood trauma, such as the death of a parent or pet, domestic turmoil, moving to a new home or starting a new school, or divorce, can all trigger a variety of symptoms similar to those of ADHD.

Part of the AAP guidelines recommend that as with other chronic conditions, treatment of ADHD requires the development of child-specific treatment plans that describe methods and goals of treatment and means of monitoring care over time, including specific plans for follow-up. Most important, ensure that a proper diagnosis is made before beginning any treatment regimen.

Once an ADHD diagnosis is made, continue to work closely with your child's doctor and other professionals to constantly evaluate how the treatment is working. This requires carefully collecting information from parents, teachers, other adults in the child's environment (for example, coaches or daycare leaders), and the child himself. If the target symptoms (inattentiveness, restlessness, and an impulsiveness abnormal for the age bracket that causes impairment in some aspect of daily life) are realistic and the lack of effectiveness using medication and behavioral therapy is clear, the primary care clinician should reassess the accuracy of the diagnosis of ADHD.

Nondrug Treatments for ADHD

For many children, medication is simply not an option. Side effects may pose a barrier, the child's nervous system simply may not benefit from the use of medication, the child may refuse to comply with taking the medication (teens especially), or the symptoms may be mild enough to warrant a nondrug approach. There are also families who begin nondrug therapy with the goal of decreasing the child's dependence on prescription medicines.

FEINGOLD DIET
Developed by Dr. Benjamin Feingold in the early 1970s, this diet, also referred to as the Feingold Program, attempts to determine which foods or food additives may trigger particular symptoms with your child. It seeks to eliminate food additives such as artificial coloring, fla-

voring, and preservatives (like BHA, BHT, and TBHQ). It is highly restrictive and may require weeks using trial and error to eliminate the right foods. With this program, it is helpful if the entire family joins in so there is no chance for the ADHD child to "find" forbidden foods. Proponents say this diet works as a first line for children diagnosed with ADHD to improve attention and behavior caused by a system overload of junk and fast food.

NATURAL SUPPLEMENTS

Many natural health–oriented doctors believe that potential causes for the modern epidemic of Attention Deficit Disorders and hyperactivity are food additives, refined sugar, poor nutrition, natural light deficiency, food allergies, or heavy metal toxicity (such as that caused by overexposure to lead, mercury, or cadmium).

Spurred by studies of nutritional deficiencies in children with ADHD, these practitioners believe that changing what goes into the child can have a profound effect on behavior. Studies cited have shown that boys diagnosed with ADHD had lower levels of the omega-3 essential fatty acid DHA, were deficient in magnesium, and had zinc levels that were only two-thirds the level of those without ADHD.

Experts recommend dietary supplementation of essential fatty acids (EFAs), including DHA/EFA supplements, fish oil, flaxseed oil, and primrose oil. Family meals should be high in the "good fats," such as olive oil, fish oil, canola oil, and flaxseed oil. All other fats should be reduced. Eliminate, or at least reduce as much as possible, trans-fats (for example, man-made hydrogenated oils). Avoid food additives and highly processed foods. Supplement your child with a high-quality multivitamin that contains trace minerals and other supplements, especially calcium, magnesium, zinc, and B vitamins.

BEHAVIORAL THERAPY

Behavioral therapy is a program that is set up to increase the frequency of acceptable behaviors and decrease the frequency of unacceptable behaviors. It is normally used with a reward and consequence structure.

There are three key aspects of shaping a child's proper social behavior through behavior modification and management techniques:

1. There are positive rewards (both verbal and concrete) for appropriate behavior.

2. There are negative consequences (taking away privileges) when poor behavior is observed.

3. There is an attempt to increase the child's desire to please his parents/caregivers by showing admiration and appreciation when good social skills are observed.

Experts recommend setting up a behavior contract with a child who has ADHD. This contract will aim to work on one behavior at a time. First, the child will identify the behavior and then the parent will assist the child in selecting an alternative, more appropriate behavior to replace the misbehavior with. All misbehaviors must be replaced with another behavior, not just simply taken away.

The atmosphere in the home greatly affects behavioral therapy. The home environment should be structured to provide support to the child with ADHD. Family and household rules should be clear and well-defined as well as consistently applied. Predictable routines often help structure time for the child with ADHD. A quiet, organized study area, free of distractions, should be set up. Constant times and routines should be established for study and review of work by the parent. The child's family responsibilities should also be well-defined, and it may be necessary to break chores or tasks into very small sequential steps. Plans should be reviewed with the child, and the child should be prepared, in advance if possible, for any changes to the ordinary routine.

ADHD Outlook

In our fast-paced world of quick fixes and one-tablet cures, the child with symptoms of ADHD often feels misplaced. His condition is one that will likely follow him into adulthood and without proper treatment may leave him with wounded self-esteem. Difficulty getting along with peers, employers, and partners in his life can have a devastating effect on emotional growth.

In addition, the parents of a child diagnosed with ADHD will face many challenges. The family as a whole must learn to adjust to the needs of the child as well as provide a nurturing environment for him to thrive. Fortunately, giant strides have been made in the ADHD treatment arsenal and more advances are being made daily. Don't be afraid to ask questions of your child's health care providers. Knowledge is key. The more the family learns about the condition and treatment options, the greater the opportunity to help the child live a happy and well-adjusted life.

2

The Antibiotic Epidemic

Your child has been up all night with a cold and a fever. As dawn breaks, you call the pediatrician for an emergency office visit. You bundle up the sick one and together you head to the doctor's office for a miserable 30-minute wait. When the doctor finally sees you, she says, "I'm sorry. It's just a cold. It needs to run its course. There isn't anything you can do except make the child more comfortable until the symptoms go away."

"What?" you exclaim. "Run its course? But, my child has an infection. I need a prescription for an antibiotic so he can feel better. So we all can get some sleep. Write me a prescription for an antibiotic. I'm not leaving here without a prescription for an antibiotic." Sound extreme? Maybe just a bit, but the fact is doctors are handing out antibiotic prescriptions by the handful to demanding parents who don't realize that they may be doing their child much more harm than good in the long run by promoting antibiotic resistance.

Antibiotic resistance is the inability of an antibiotic to effectively shut down invading bacteria. The overuse of antibiotics in certain children's infections contributes to this potentially life-threatening problem. At this time, we have only a limited arsenal of antibiotics. What happens when the antibiotics we have no longer control the bacteria causing an infection?

How Antibiotics Work

To learn how dangerous antibiotic overuse can be, it is helpful to learn just how antibiotics do their job. The first fact to remember is that antibiotics have absolutely no effect on viruses. In addition, viruses cause nearly all childhood colds and coughs, as well as many ear infections.

An antibiotic may mount an attack on infection-causing bacteria in several ways. It can erode the cell wall of the bacteria, destroying the contents before they can cause damage. It can also upset the essential processes within the bacterial cell, such as protein synthesis and energy production, rendering the bacteria useless.

Your doctor will make the determination of whether or not an antibiotic is warranted for your child's illness. This can be done in several ways. The most effective way is by taking a culture and testing it for offending bacteria. For example, a doctor may take a swab and rub it along the back of the throat when strep throat is suspected. Often, though, the doctor is familiar with the type of bacterial infection, such as a urinary tract infection or ear infection, and can prescribe medicine specific for that type. Other factors, like the cost of medication for those without insurance or a more convenient (and more likely to be followed) dosing schedule are also often taken into account.

An important part of how well antibiotics work for your child is knowing how to give them properly. Always double-check with your pharmacist before heading home with the medicine. Some children's antibiotics must be refrigerated to retain their potency; with others, refrigeration isn't necessary.

Liquid antibiotics are usually dispensed with a "shake well" label. This is to ensure that all of the medication hasn't settled to the bottom and to prevent the first doses from being nothing but colored water.

Having food on the stomach is an important consideration for some antibiotics. For others, it doesn't matter. Some types of food, like dairy products or milk, may interfere with the effectiveness of some antibiotics. Ask your pharmacist to be sure.

Even if your child begins to feel better, please, please, continue the full course of antibiotics. Stopping before the infection is completely cleared can give bacteria time to mutate and become more resistant to the antibiotic being given. The next time this type of infection strikes, the antibiotic may not work as well. Also, be sure to toss out any leftover antibiotics. Don't save a partial course of therapy for another time when the child may not feel well.

Types of Antibiotics

There are more than one hundred different antibiotics on the market today. These are classified according to the range of bacteria they fight best. There are narrow-spectrum antibiotics, which are effective against only a few types of bacteria, and broad-spectrum antibiotics, which can eliminate a wide range of bacteria. Antibiotics can be further divided into classes based on the type of bacteria they target.

CLASSES OF ANTIBIOTICS AND COMMON BRAND NAMES
■ **Penicillins (and amoxicillins)**
Common brand names: PenVK, Veetids, Beepen-VK, Amoxil, Polymox, and Wymox.

Common illnesses penicillins are prescribed for include dental infections, ear infections, respiratory tract infections, urinary tract infections, and skin infections.

Augmentin, also in the penicillin family, is a product containing amoxicillin and clavulanic acid. It is a potent combination of penicillin and a beta-lactamase inhibitor to give the antibiotic extra protection from bacterial enzymes until it has time to do its job.

A Drug Lady Reminder

Severe penicillin allergies occur in only three to five percent of the population. Infants and young children are most at risk with the first several doses of the medicine. Look for signs of swelling around the face and throat, hives, and rash. Most reactions are mild, however a true allergic reaction can turn quickly to anaphylactic shock (see Anaphylactic Shock, pg. 138), so prompt medical attention is required.

■ Cephalosporins

Common brand names: Keflex (cephalexin), Ceclor (cefaclor), Duricef (cefadroxil), Suprax (cefixime), Cefzil (cefprozil), and Ceftin (cefuroxime).

These antibiotics are used to treat infections in the ears, nose, throat, lungs, sinuses, and skin. A diagnosis of strep throat, staph infections, tonsillitis, or bronchitis prompts use of this class of drugs.

■ Tetracyclines (and doxycyclines)

Common brand names: Sumycin, Doryx (doxycycline), and Vibramycin (doxycycline).

These antibiotics are used to treat acne, eye infections, pneumonia, and urinary tract infections.

■ Macrolides

Common brand names: E-mycin, Ery-C, Ery-Tab (erythromycin), Biaxin (clarithromycin), and Zithromax (azithromycin).

These drugs are prescribed for many types of infections caused

A Drug Lady Reminder

A child experiencing a reaction to sulfa medication will generally get a red, itchy rash. The medicine should be stopped right away and the doctor called for a substitute. Typically, the reaction is mild, but more severe reactions can lead to anaphylactic shock (see Anaphylactic Shock, pg. 138) and prompt medical attention is required. Another caution with sulfa-based medications is to avoid sun exposure while the medication is being taken. Nasty burns can result from only a short time in the sun (see Sun-Sensitive Medications, pg. 121).

by bacteria, including strep throat, sinus infections, ear infections, pneumonia, bronchitis, tonsillitis, and urinary tract infections.

■ Sulfonamides

Common brand names: Bactrim (sulfamethoxazole/trimethoprim) and Gantrisin (sulfisoxazole).

These are also referred to as the "sulfa" drugs. They are used to treat urinary tract infections, ear or eye infections, bronchitis, meningitis, and traveler's diarrhea.

■ Aminoglycosides

Common brand names: Garamycin (gentamicin), Tobrex (tobramycin), Amikin (amikacin) and Mycifradin (neomycin).

These powerful antibiotics are used to treat intestinal infections and tuberculosis, or used topically to treat eye infections. *Pseudomonas*, *Acinetobacter*, and *Enterobacter* are strains of bacteria that can successfully be fought with aminoglycosides.

A Drug Lady Reminder

Research suggests that antibiotics in the fluorquinolone class may cause bone development problems in children and teenagers. These are Cipro (ciprofloxacin), Trovan (trovafloxin), Levaquin (levofloxacin), Noroxin (norfloxacin), and Floxin (ofloxacin). Package insert information states, "Infants, children, teenagers, pregnant women, and women who are breastfeeding should not take this medicine unless directed to do so by a physician."

■ Fluorquinolones

Common brand names: Cipro (ciprofloxacin), Trovan (trovafloxin), Levaquin (levofloxacin), Noroxin (norfloxacin), and Floxin (ofloxacin).

Cipro (ciprofloxacin) has been in the news as the drug to treat anthrax (see Bioterrorism and Your Child, pg. 33). Other common conditions treated with this class of antibiotics are urinary tract infections; infections of the skin, bones, and joints; ear infections; pneumonia; bronchitis; tuberculosis; infections affecting immune-compromised individuals, and some sexually transmitted diseases.

The Overuse of Antibiotics

The U.S. government estimates that over 50 million of the antibiotic prescriptions written each year are unnecessary. This means that nearly 50 million individuals are taking medicine that is unlikely to make them any better and may, in fact, greatly increase the chance that the next time they get sick, an antibiotic will not work.

Studies show that 46 percent of patients who visit the doctor for a cold (caused by a virus) will receive a prescription for an antibiotic, even when the doctor is aware that no other condition, other than the common cold or sinusitis is present. Another study found that more than 80 percent of children's middle ear infections would clear up on their own without using an antibiotic.

Newer drugs of the broad-spectrum variety are prescribed 53 percent of the time. A shift from the older narrow-spectrum antibiotics, like penicillins, that destroy more specific strains of bacteria to the broader-spectrum varieties that destroy everything is bringing antibiotic resistance to potentially crisis levels. There are several reasons for this overprescribing trend. One explanation is the tremendous power of direct-to-consumer advertising. A patient sees a particular medicine on television or in print media and demands that the doctor write a prescription for it. Other patients have certain expectations when they go into a doctor's office with an infection. They may feel that they aren't being treated if there is no antibiotic prescription in their hand when they leave.

The Dangers of Antibiotic Resistance

Antibiotic resistance may also be referred to as drug resistance, as in "drug resistant bacteria." Bacteria that cause illness have the ability to change or mutate as part of their survival mechanism. When they are constantly exposed to an agent, like an antibiotic, trying to wipe them out, they change, or become resistant. This mutation is survival of the fittest for bacteria strains. Unfortunately, this change makes them immune or resistant to the effects of that antibiotic the next time it is given. The bacteria now have free rein to multiply without restraint. While this is good news for the bacteria, it is not good news when your child's body is trying to fight a raging infection. As resistance increases, the antibiotic weapons supply dwindles.

By July 2004, in some parts of the United States, over 60 percent of the bacteria responsible for childhood infections ranging from those of the middle ear to meningitis may be resistant to both penicillin and erythromycin. This isn't science fiction, but information from a research study at Harvard University School of Public Health published in *Nature Medicine* on March 10, 2003. Using a mathematical model, these scientists showed how the common bacteria *Streptococcus pneumoniae* would develop resistant strains against what has always been the backbone of the antibiotic cache. *Streptococcus pneumoniae* bacteria are to blame for most ear infections, sinus infections, and bacterial meningitis.

If antibiotic resistance continues at the rate of today, we are in grave danger of losing the battle with chronic infections and for those whose immune system is already compromised. Super germs have a chance to develop unchecked by any methods we have at hand. The Centers for Disease Control calls antibiotic resistance "one of the world's most pressing public health problems."

Stopping Antibiotic Resistance

The good news is that studies show the trend toward overprescribing of antibiotics has slowed dramatically. The bad news is that it may already be too late. The overuse of broad-spectrum antibiotics may have caused resistance to many of the antibiotics we've depended on since the 1930s.

The Food and Drug Administration (FDA) and your pharmacist are getting involved in trying to avert this potential health crisis. A new labeling system alerts the pharmacist when a new antibiotic is prescribed, so she can counsel the patient "that antibacterial drugs, including the antibacterial drug product prescribed, should only be used to treat bacterial infections and that they do not treat viruses." In addition, "when an antibacterial drug is prescribed to treat a bacterial infection, patients should be told that although it is common to feel better early in the course of therapy, the medication should be taken exactly as directed." With this new labeling system, the FDA hopes to reduce the "inappropriate prescribing of antibiotics to children and adults for common ailments such as ear infections and chronic coughs."

With every doctor visit, it is important to remember that antibiotics aren't for all infections, so don't press the doctor to write a prescription for a medicine your child may not need.

Be an informed parent. Ask if the illness is caused by a bacteria or virus. Ask the doctor and the pharmacist about the specific antibiotic prescribed for your child. Is it a broad- or narrow-spectrum antibiotic? Is it really necessary?

Don't forget that when your child is feeling better after only three days of the medicine, continue to give it for the full ten to 14 days to ensure that the bacteria causing the infection are completely and totally wiped out.

3

Bioterrorism and Your Child

Within the past few years, we've been forced to address issues that we hoped would never impact our lives or those of our families. Bioterrorism, or the use of biological products as a weapon, is now something we must not only address, but for our family's sake, we must take steps to prepare for as well.

Preparing for Bioterrorism

No one likes to consider the possibility of a bioterrorism attack that would put families at risk. However, with the volatility of current events, it is indeed a possibility. It is important to be prepared—both mentally and physically. While there is no absolute method of preparation for a bioterrorism attack, there are certain things you can do as a parent and as a family to ensure your family is as safe as possible.

Number one, have a plan. Talk with your family and educate everyone on the importance of living life normally, but having in the back of their minds what to do in case of an emergency. An important part of the plan is designating rally points for the family. Because your family is not together 24 hours a day, you need to consider how you would find each other in a disaster. Rally points, or meeting locations, should be identified for the places where the family most commonly frequents. For example, if a crisis occurs at school, predetermine a location where you and your family would meet.

The American Academy of Pediatrics (AAP) recommends putting together an extensive "Family Readiness Kit" to ensure the family is prepared in the event of a bioterrorism attack or any other type of disaster. Items in this kit would include:

- A battery-powered radio and flash light

- Extra batteries

- A family first-aid kit

- A one-month supply of essential prescription medications if the pharmacy is unavailable

- Credit cards and cash

- Car keys

- Personal identification for all family members

- Signal flares

- A whistle

- A map of the area

- Three gallons of water per person

- Chlorine bleach (for sanitizing drinking water)

- Special needs items for infants/babies

- Sunscreen and insect repellant for warm climates

- Automatic can openers/bottle openers

■ Cups, plates, and utensils

■ Plastic garbage bags

■ Blankets or sleeping bags

■ A change of clothing and sturdy shoes for all members of the family

Keep these essentials in a duffle bag or clearly labeled backpack and store in an easily accessible place, like the basement or garage.

Bioterrorism Dangers

ANTHRAX

What Is Anthrax?

Anthrax is a disease caused by the spore-forming bacteria called *Bacillus anthracis*. This disease is highly dangerous because the spores are relatively easy to spread and cultivate, creating the potential for large-scale distribution by air. There are actually two different forms of anthrax, causing three different patterns of illness. Cutaneous anthrax involves the skin and the gastrointenstinal tract, while inhalation anthrax affects the lungs.

The Symptoms of Anthrax

Cutaneous anthrax of the skin occurs after the bacteria has come in contact with areas of the skin that have cuts or abrasions. Usually within two weeks, an itchy skin lesion develops that is similar to an insect bite. This lesion may later blister and then break down, resulting in a black ulcer, which is usually painless. Swelling occurs around the ulcer. The lymph nodes may also swell and become tender. A scab is often formed that then dries and falls off within two weeks. In 20 percent of individuals, the infection may spread through the bloodstream and become fatal. However, in most individuals who receive appropriate medical treatment, death from this form of cutaneous anthrax is rare.

The gastrointestinal form of cutaneous anthrax occurs when meat contaminated with anthrax spores is eaten. This disease usually develops within one week and can affect the upper portion of the gastrointestinal tract (mouth and esophagus) or the intestines and colon. Symptoms include nausea and vomiting (which may include blood), loss of appetite, and bloody diarrhea. Infection in both of these areas may result in spread of the infection by the bloodstream and can result in death.

The inhalation form of anthrax develops when anthrax spores enter the lungs. A person may have spores in the nasal passages, which indicates exposure, but may never come down with symptoms of the disease. In fact, antibiotic therapy following known or suspected exposure can help prevent anthrax. In order for a person to develop the actual disease, the spores must germinate or begin to grow and release toxins. This process may take several days, or even up to two months to occur. The spores move to the lymph nodes, resulting in hemorrhage, swelling, and tissue death. The main form of inhalation anthrax includes infection of the lymph nodes in the chest, also called hemorrhagic mediastinitis. Up to half of affected individuals may also have hemorrhagic meningitis. There are usually two stages of inhalation anthrax: The first stage can last from hours to a few days and is similar to a flu-like illness with fever, headache, cough, shortness of breath, and chest pain. The second stage often develops suddenly and is notable for shortness of breath, fever, and body system shock. This second stage is fatal in up to 90 percent of individuals because of the buildup of toxins.

Emergency Response

Anthrax is a very dangerous tool for bioterrorists. In theory, one kilogram of anthrax could kill 10,000 people. Fortunately, technical difficulties with preparing the spores in a sufficiently fine powder would probably limit actual deaths to a fraction of this.

For individuals who have been truly exposed to anthrax (but have no signs and symptoms of the disease), preventive antibiotics may be offered, such as ciprofloxacin, penicillin, or doxycycline, depending on the particular strain of anthrax.

A vaccination has also been developed and is given in a six-dose series. This vaccine is mandated for all U.S. military personnel. It is currently not available, nor is it recommended, for use in the general public.

Anthrax is not transmitted from person to person. Household contacts of individuals with anthrax do not need antibiotics unless they have also been exposed to the same source of anthrax. Even if you are unaware of a particular exposure to anthrax, if anyone in the family develops skin lesions or flu-like symptoms, you should contact the doctor. While there are many illnesses with similar symptoms, your child will need a medical evaluation to sort out which illness is causing his symptoms.

SMALLPOX

What Is Smallpox?

Smallpox is caused by a virus called *variola*, in the same family as the chicken pox virus (*varicella*). Symptoms are similar to chicken pox. The features that distinguish smallpox from chicken pox are:

■ Chicken pox has a fever that begins at the same time the skin rash appears, while the smallpox fever is typically high (over 101° F) and appears two to four days before the skin rash appears.

■ Severe stomach pain, back pain, and delirium occur before the smallpox rash appears; these are not present before the chicken pox rash appears.

■ The rash of chicken pox usually starts on the scalp; with smallpox, the lesions appear first on the face, mouth, throat, and forearms.

Smallpox is transmitted by face-to-face contact with respiratory water droplets, such as coughs or sneezes, of an infected person. Smallpox also can be spread through direct contact with infected bodily fluids or contaminated objects such as bedding or clothing. Young children and unvaccinated individuals are at highest risk if an outbreak occurs. Unfortunately, there is no cure for smallpox. Smallpox response teams, made up of vaccinated health care professionals, will be the front line to provide services in case of a smallpox outbreak.

The Symptoms of Smallpox

Flu-like symptoms begin approximately two weeks after exposure to the virus. A high fever, severe headache, backache, vomiting, diarrhea, and fatigue are first noticed; then sores develop in the mouth and throat. Skin lesions (raised and pink bumps) then appear on the body. The rash begins on the face and spreads down the body. The bumps fill with pus and crust over on the eighth or ninth day after first symptoms.

A person with smallpox is sometimes contagious with onset of fever (the prodrome phase, which occurs two to four days before the rash), but the person becomes most contagious with the onset of rash. At this stage, the infected person is usually very sick. The infected person is contagious until the last smallpox scab falls off.

Emergency Response

Smallpox is considered a Category A (high-priority) agent for a bioterrorist attack because it can easily be spread from person to person in powder form or contaminated dirt. It would take no more than 50 to one hundred cases to cause legitimate concern on an international level. Twenty to 30 percent of unvaccinated individuals will die from exposure to smallpox, while those surviving typically suffer permanent scarring and/or loss of eyesight.

The best prevention is vaccination. If given within one to four days after exposure, it may prevent the illness or decrease severity of the outbreak. The vaccine is not made from the smallpox virus, but from a relative called vaccina. It's not an injection of the virus, but rather the skin is pricked with a two-pronged needle dipped in the vaccine. This vaccine type of virus is very contagious. When vaccinated, the child's vaccination site must be carefully protected from injury, scratching, and traumas to prevent spread of this virus to others. Long-sleeved shirts and a frequently changed heavy bandage are good choices until the site heals.

It is recommended that children younger than 18 years of age who are not exposed to smallpox avoid the vaccination, as well as any child younger than 12 months of age. Dangers of possible vaccine infections and complications that may arise outweigh the risks at this time. Hospital, medical, and emergency personnel are advised to be vaccinated. If there is a smallpox attack, officials are likely to order mass inoculations for all adults and children. If someone were diagnosed with smallpox, they (and all other face-to-face contacts) would need to be isolated immediately.

RADIATION

What Is Radiation Sickness?

In the event of a nuclear accident, like a nuclear power plant explosion or crash of a transport vehicle, or intentional nuclear catastrophe, it is important to be prepared for radiation disasters. Any of these events could occur unintentionally or as an act of terrorism. There are two types of radiation: the nonionizing variety that consists of radio waves, microwaves, and light waves, and the ionizing variety of X rays, gamma rays, and atomic particles.

Radiation sickness occurs when there is exposure to high doses of ionizing radiation that causes tissue damage and death. If exposure to radiation is in small doses over a long period of time, the body responds by contracting various cancers and ages prematurely. Children are at higher risk because they are growing more rapidly; there are more cells dividing and a greater opportunity for radiation to disrupt the process.

Radiation sickness is also called radiation poisoning. If the dose is fatal, death usually occurs within two months. For exposure to large amounts of radiation (acute exposure), the symptoms depend on how much was absorbed and the rate at which it was absorbed:

- 100 rads total body exposure = radiation sickness

- 400 rads total body exposure = radiation sickness and death in 50 percent of cases

- 100,000 rads = immediate unconsciousness and death within one hour

For comparison of the usual rate of exposure, most people receive about three-tenths of a rad every year from natural background sources of radiation (mostly radon) found in the soil and air we breathe.

The Symptoms of Radiation Sickness
The earliest symptoms of radiation sickness are nausea, fatigue, vomiting, and diarrhea; however it may take days or weeks after exposure

before these appear. Skin burns with redness and blistering may be apparent. Open sores and sloughing of the skin may occur. Hair loss; hemorrhaging of the nose, mouth, and gums; swelling of the mouth and throat; and general loss of energy may follow.

Emergency Response

The AAP recommends immediate access to potassium iodide by parents, schools, and day-care centers within a ten mile radius of nuclear power plants. Potassium iodide is of proven value for protection against thyroid cancer in the case of a radiation emergency, but must be given before or soon after exposure to radioiodines. Brands approved by the FDA include Thyro-Block (MedPointe, Inc.), IOSTAT (Anbex, Inc.), and Thyro-Safe (Recip US).

Unfortunately, potassium iodide has no affect on other radiation-induced side effects like nausea, vomiting, hair loss, or even other cancers. The child's doctor may order medications to ease nausea and pain. Blood counts may be ordered to assess the cell damage and determine further treatment.

If a radiation disaster should occur, parents are urged to pay close attention to recommendations from Public Health Services. Do not remain in the area where exposure occurred. Do not remain in exposed clothing. Do not apply creams or ointments to exposed skin.

4

Childhood Immunizations: Are They Safe and Effective Today?

Immunizations and Why They Are Important

From the first hepatitis B shot your newborn receives in the hospital to the seemingly endless series of immunizations required for school, parents can feel helpless and overwhelmed at the prospect of what is being done to their child. Diphtheria, pertussis (whooping cough), tetanus (lockjaw), *Haemophilus influenzae* type b, measles, mumps, rubella, chicken pox, polio, and hepatitis B—the parade can seem to be endless. Parents wonder: Is the shot necessary? Will it hurt my child? What should I expect? The best way to conquer these fears is to become informed about the potential risks and proven benefits of immunizations. Learn what the vaccine protects your child from and what side effects (if any) to expect.

An immunization is a method of preventing the spread of a contagious disease by introducing a minute amount of a foreign substance (an antigen) into the body. Antigens can be bacterial, viral or formed from toxins. The body begins to produce antibodies that serve as protection in case it is exposed to the live virus, bacteria, or toxin during an outbreak. So instead of waiting until a deadly epidemic strikes and attempting to treat it, the population as a whole is protected from ever coming down with the disease.

Vaccinations today provide protection from over 11 potentially deadly infections. Just one example is measles. In developing countries that don't immunize, measles kills nearly one million children a year. In the United States, the MMR vaccine has brought the total number of cases of measles to fewer than one hundred. The number of children who come down with preventable diseases is down 99 percent since 1972.

Immunization Concerns

In one survey, 80 percent of new parents did not know which immunizations their child needed or what the shot protected them from. In addition, many parents have concerns over vaccination safety and whether vaccinations are really necessary. Here are some common questions and answers.

ARE ALL VACCINES SAFE?

Unfortunately, all vaccines, like any drugs, have the potential for side effects or adverse reactions in a child. (See vaccination side effects, pg. 47.) Over 100 million vaccinations are given in the United States every year. Typically, the reactions are mild and short-lived; however, there are rare cases when problems that are more serious are noted. Before vaccines are licensed, the Food and Drug Administration (FDA) requires they be extensively tested to ensure safety. This process can take ten years or longer.

No parent wants to expose their child to unnecessary risks, so to make the best decision for your child, it is important to be informed.

In almost every instance, the benefits of childhood immunizations far outweigh the potential risks. Devastating diseases, like polio and smallpox, have been virtually eradicated from a parent's worry list. Measles, whooping cough, and diphtheria are diseases we see rarely. In addition to the diseases themselves, unvaccinated children are at risk from pneumonia caused by measles, meningitis (swelling of the lining of the brain) caused by Hib (a severe bacterial infection), bloodstream infections caused by pneumococcus, deafness caused by mumps, and liver cancer caused by hepatitis B virus.

CAN IMMUNIZATIONS WEAKEN MY CHILD'S IMMUNE SYSTEM?
Many parents worry that the large battery of shots given to their young child will damage his immune system. In fact, today's vaccines contain smaller amounts of the antigens required to produce antibodies. In the past, the polio vaccine used the actual live virus, and there was the possibility of transmitting the disease from the vaccine, but today it has been largely replaced with an inactivated polio vaccine.

IS THERE A CONNECTION BETWEEN AUTISM AND THE MMR VACCINE?
There are many studies underway, and to date, there is no scientific evidence to show that vaccines cause autism. The Institute of Medicine's Immunization Safety Review Committee recently examined studies about the health effects of the Measles-Mumps-Rubella (MMR) vaccine in young children and found that the evidence showed no contributory relationship between MMR vaccine and autistic spectrum disorders.

IS IT TRUE THAT MY CHILD CAN GET MERCURY POISONING FROM HIS SHOTS?

Before 1999, there were cases of higher than normal mercury levels in infants receiving vaccines with the preservative thimerosal. Since that time, however, the FDA has required all vaccines to be thimerosal-free. There should be no danger of mercury from any vaccines given today.

Reacting to Problems Caused by Immunizations

There is always a small possibility that your child may react to a particular vaccination. If your recently immunized child is acting unusual, call a doctor. If your child is having a severe reaction (see Anaphylactic Shock, pg. 138), get her to a doctor right away. After any reaction, tell your doctor what happened, the date and time it happened, and when the vaccination was given. Your health care provider is required to fill out a VAERS. VAERS is the Vaccine Adverse Events Reporting System. Ask your doctor, nurse, or health department to file a VAERS form, or call VAERS yourself at 1-800-822-7967.

VAERS was established in 1990. Once a vaccine is in use, the Centers for Disease Control (CDC) and the FDA monitor its side effects through VAERS. Any hint of a problem with a vaccine prompts further investigations by the CDC and FDA. If researchers find a vaccine may be causing a side effect, the CDC and FDA will initiate actions appropriate to the nature of the problem. This may include the changing of vaccine labels or packaging, distributing safety alerts, inspecting manufacturers' facilities and records, withdrawing recommendations for the use of the vaccine, or revoking the vaccine's license.

The National Vaccine Injury Compensation Program (VICP) ensures an adequate supply of vaccines, stabilizes vaccine costs, and establishes and maintains an accessible and efficient forum for individuals thought to be injured by childhood vaccines. Settlements are based on the list of adverse events caused by vaccines. You can visit their website at www.hrsa.gov/osp/vicp for more information.

Vaccination Types and Side Effects

Following is a roundup from the CDC of the diseases a particular vaccination is aimed at preventing, along with the side effects, both common and rare, associated with those vaccinations.

DIPHTHERIA, PERTUSSIS, AND TETANUS
Vaccines: DPT and DPaT

1. Mild problems (common):

   - Fever (up to about one child in four)
   - Redness or swelling where the shot was given (up to about one child in four)
   - Soreness or tenderness where the shot was given (up to about one child in four)

These problems occur more often after the fourth and fifth doses of the DPaT series than after earlier doses. Sometimes the fourth or fifth dose of the DPaT vaccine is followed by swelling of the entire arm or leg in which the shot was given, for one to seven days (up to about one child in thirty).

2. Mild problems (less common):

- Fussiness (up to about one child in three)
- Tiredness or poor appetite (up to about one child in ten)
- Vomiting (up to about one child in 50)

These problems generally occur one to three days after the shot.

3. Moderate problems (uncommon):

- Seizure (jerking or staring) (up to about one child in 14,000)
- Nonstop crying, for three hours or more (up to about one child in 1,000)
- High fever, over 105°F (up to about one child in 16,000)

4. Severe problems (very rare):

- Serious allergic reaction (less than one out of a million doses)
- Long-term seizures, coma, or lowered consciousness (so rare that it is difficult to tell if they are caused by the vaccine)
- Permanent brain damage (so rare that it is difficult to tell if they are caused by the vaccine)

HEPATITIS B

1. Mild problems:

- Soreness where the shot was given, lasting a day or two (up to about one child or adolescent in 11, and up to about one adult in four)
- Mild to moderate fever (up to about one child or adolescent in 14 and one adult out of one hundred)

2. Severe problems:

- Serious allergic reaction (very rare)

HAEMOPHILUS INFLUENZAE TYPE B (HIB)
Vaccine: Hib

1. Mild problems:

   ■ Redness, warmth, or swelling where the shot was given (up to one child in four)
   ■ Fever over 101°F (up to one child in 20)

If these problems happen, they usually start within a day of the vaccination. They may last two to three days.

MEASLES, MUMPS, AND RUBELLA
Vaccine: MMR

1. Mild problems:

   ■ Fever (up to one child in six)
   ■ Mild rash (about one child in 20)
   ■ Swelling of glands in the cheeks or neck (rare)

If these problems occur, it is usually within seven to 12 days after the shot. They occur less often after the second dose.

2. Moderate problems:

   ■ Seizure (jerking or staring) caused by fever (about one out of 3,000 doses)
   ■ Temporary pain and stiffness in the joints, mostly in teenage or adult women (up to one in four)
   ■ Temporary low platelet count, which can cause a bleeding disorder (about one out of 30,000 doses)

3. Severe problems (very rare):

- Serious allergic reaction (less than one out of a million doses)
- Several other severe problems have been known to occur after a child gets MMR vaccine. However, this happens so rarely, experts cannot be sure whether the vaccine causes them or not. These include deafness, long-term seizures, coma, or lowered consciousness, and permanent brain damage

STREPTOCOCCUS PNEUMONIAE

Vaccine: Pneumococcal conjugate vaccine

In studies involving nearly 60,000 doses, pneumococcal conjugate vaccine was associated with only mild reactions:

- Up to about one infant in four had redness, tenderness, or swelling where the shot was administered

- Up to about one in three had a fever of over 100.4°F, and up to about one in fifty had a higher fever (over 102.2°F)

- Some children also became fussy or drowsy, or had a loss of appetite

So far, no moderate or severe reactions have been associated with this vaccine.

POLIO

Vaccines: IPV or OPV

There are two kinds of polio vaccine: IPV (inactivated polio vaccine), which is the shot recommended in the United States today, and a live, oral polio vaccine (OPV). Until recently, OPV was recommended for most children in the United States. OPV helped us rid the country of polio, and it is still used in many parts of the world. Both vaccines give immunity to polio, but OPV is better at keeping the disease from spreading to other people. However, for a few people (about one in 2.4 million), OPV actually causes polio. Since the risk of getting polio in the United States is now extremely low, experts believe that using OPV is no longer worth the slight risk, except in limited circumstances. IPV does not cause polio.

Some people who get IPV get a sore spot where the shot was given. The vaccine used today is not known to cause any serious problems.

VARICELLA (CHICKEN POX)

1. Mild problems:

   - Soreness or swelling where the shot was given (about one child in five and up to one adolescent and adult in three)
   - Fever (one person in ten or less)
   - Mild rash up to a month after vaccination (one person in 20 or less). It is possible for these people to infect other members of their household, but this is extremely rare

2. Moderate problems:

   - Seizure (jerking or staring) caused by fever (less than one person in 1,000)

3. Severe problems:

   - Pneumonia (very rare)
   - Other serious problems, including severe brain reactions and low blood count, have been reported after a chicken pox vaccination. These happen so rarely experts cannot tell whether the vaccine causes them or not

A Drug Lady Reminder

Discomfort and fever associated with vaccines can be treated at home with Children's Tylenol (acetaminophen) or Motrin (ibuprofen). Check with your child's doctor about which to use after their particular series of shots.

Immunization Regulations

According to the CDC National Vaccine Program Office, each state has vaccination (immunization) requirements, sometimes called "school laws," which must be met before a child may enter school. These may include vaccination against diphtheria, pertussis (whooping cough), tetanus (lockjaw), *Haemophilus influenzae* type b, measles, mumps, rubella, polio, and hepatitis B. Some states have added varicella (chicken pox) vaccination to the list of required vaccines. Smallpox vaccination was once required, but the disease has been so successfully eradicated that this vaccination is no longer needed. In most states, a parent must bring written proof of a child's immunizations from the health care provider or clinic at the time of school registration. If a required vaccination has not been obtained, and there is no health condition or religious objection preventing immunization, the child must receive the vaccinations before they can enroll for school.

These required vaccinations don't only protect the children in a classroom. They protect the teachers, parent volunteers, visiting grandparents, and everyone else who enters the classroom or provides services to the school. The blanket of protection provided by rubella (German measles) vaccination is especially important for women who are pregnant. Rubella can cause serious damage to the developing fetus, including deafness, blindness, heart disease, brain damage, or other serious problems, such as miscarriage.

You can find out what the requirements for vaccinations are in your state at http://www.cdc.gov/od/nvpo/law.htm.

Immunization Schedule

Recommended Childhood and Adolescent Immunization Schedule in the United States

	Birth	1 month	2 months	4 months	6 months	12 months	15 months	18 months	24 months	4-6years	11-12 years	13-18 years
Hepatitis B	A	B	B	B	C	C	C					
DPT			D	E	F		G	G		H	Z	
H. Influenza Type b			I	J	K	L	L					
Inactived Poliovirus			M	N	O	O	O	O		P		
MMR						Q	Q			R		
Varicella						S	S	S				
Pneumococcal		T	U	V	W	W						
Hepatitis A*									X	X	X	X
Influenza*					Y	Y	Y	Y	Y	Y	Y	Y

*For selected populations.

HEPATITIS B

A. First Dose: Birth to two months. Children whose mothers are hepatitis B surface antigen positive or whose hepatitis B surface antigen status is unknown should get this dose within 12 hours of birth. All infants should receive the first dose of hepatitis B vaccine soon after birth and before hospital discharge. The first dose may also be given by age two months if the infant's mother is hepatitis B surface antigen negative.

B. Second Dose: One to four months, but at least four weeks after the first dose except for combination vaccines, which cannot be administered before age six weeks.

C. Third Dose: Six to 18 months, but at least 16 weeks after the first dose and at least eight weeks after the second dose. The last dose in the vaccination series (third or fourth dose) should not be administered before age six months.

DPT—DIPHTHERIA, TETANUS, PERTUSSIS

D. First Dose: Two months.

E. Second Dose: Four months.

F. Third Dose: Six months.

G. Fourth Dose: Fifteen to 18 months. The fourth dose of DPaT may be administered as early as age 12 months, provided six months have elapsed since the third dose and the child is unlikely to return at age 15 to 18 months.

H. Fifth Dose: Four to six years.

Z. Continuing Dose: Td booster recommended at age 11 to 12 years if at least five years have elapsed since the last dose of tetanus and diphtheria toxoid-containing vaccine. Subsequent routine Td boosters are recommended every ten years.

HAEMOPHILUS INFLUENZAE TYPE B (HIB)

I. First Dose: Two months.

J. Second Dose: Four months.

K. **Third Dose:** Six months. If PRP-OMP (Pedvax HIB ® or Com-Vax ® [Merck]) is administered at ages two and four months, a dose at age six months is not required.

L. **Fourth Dose:** Twelve to 15 months.

INACTIVATED POLIOVIRUS

M. **First Dose:** Two months.

N. **Second Dose:** Four months.

O. **Third Dose:** Six to 18 months.

P. **Fourth Dose:** Four to six years.

MMR—MEASLES, MUMPS, RUBELLA

Q. **First Dose:** Twelve to 15 months.

R. **Second Dose:** Four to six years. The second dose of MMR is recommended routinely at age four to six years but may be administered during any visit, provided at least four weeks have elapsed since the first dose and that both doses are administered beginning at or after age 12 months. Those who have not previously received the second dose should complete the schedule by the time they are 11 to 12 years old.

VARICELLA (CHICKEN POX)

S. **Varicella vaccination:** Twelve to 18 months. Varicella vaccine is recommended at any visit at or after age 12 months for susceptible children—for example, those who lack a reliable history of chicken pox. Susceptible persons 13 years of age or older should receive two doses, given at least four weeks apart.

PNEUMOCOCCAL CONJUGATE VACCINE

T. First Dose: Two months.

U. Second Dose: Four months.

V. Third Dose: Six months.

W. Fourth Dose: Twelve to 15 months. The heptavalent pneumococcal conjugate vaccine (PCV) is recommended for all children aged two to 23 months. It is also recommended for certain children aged 24 to 59 months.

HEPATITIS A

X. The hepatitis A series may be given to children two years of age or older. Hepatitis A vaccine is recommended for use in selected states and regions, and for certain high-risk groups; consult your local public health authority to see if your state or region recommends this vaccination. Children and adolescents in these states, regions, and high-risk groups who have not been immunized against hepatitis A can begin the hepatitis A vaccination series during any visit. The two doses in the series should be administered at least six months apart.

INFLUENZA

Y. Influenza vaccine is recommended annually for children six months of age or older with certain risk factors, including but not limited to asthma, cardiac disease, sickle cell disease, HIV, and diabetes. It is also recommended for household members of persons in groups at high risk, and can be administered to all others wishing to obtain immunity.

In addition, healthy children age six to twenty-three months are encouraged to receive influenza vaccine if feasible because children in this age group are at substantially increased risk for influenza-related hospitalizations. Children twelve years of age or younger should receive vaccine in a dosage appropriate for their age. Children eight years of age or younger who are receiving influenza vaccine for the first time should receive two doses separated by at least four weeks.

CATCH-UP VACCINATIONS

Certain age groups require special care when receiving vaccines not previously given. These include:

- For the hepatitis B series, anybody 24 months and older.

- For the second dose of MMR, anybody 11 or 12 years old or older.

- For varicella vaccine, anybody 24 months and older.

- For pneumococcal conjugate vaccine, anybody 24 months through 59 months.

A preadolescent assessment is recommended at 11 to 12 years.

5

Avoiding Accidental Overdose

Giving medications is one of the all-time challenges parents must face. It is bad enough that your little angel is sick. Now you must force them to take something so vile that they look at you in horror when you simply pick up the bottle. Never mind that you now must try to put it into a scary contraption to shoot it quickly in their mouths. Do we really think that if we do it fast enough they won't notice?

According to the National Center for Health Statistics, over six million children each year have had illnesses for which they took prescription medicines for at least three months. That doesn't even count all of the acute conditions like earaches and sore throats that require medication. Children's smaller systems can put them at increased risk for accidental overdose. Taking medicines improperly or not at all can increase the time the child stays ill.

As a parent, you can do your part by double-checking dosages given at home as well as those prescribed by the doctor and filled by the pharmacist. A little extra diligence can mean a great deal for your child's health. Following are real questions from parents who had concerns about giving medicines to their children.

Measuring Medicines

At the drugstore I was offered a plastic syringe and a plastic spoon for giving my two year old his medicine. Unfortunately, he will only take medicine from "his" special spoon at home. Is it okay to give him his medicine this way?

If your child will only take medicine from "his" spoon, wonderful. Should you measure it in "his" spoon? No way. Dosing instruments from the pharmacy measure the medicine in milliliters, teaspoonfuls, ounces, and tablespoonfuls. It is always very important to use these for the first measurement instead of a household spoon because a household spoon can vary in size as much as 50 percent! So measure first, then administer with "his" spoon.

Because children are small and their doses are so precise, it is important that your child's dose be as accurate as possible. Measuring devices for children's medicines come in all shapes and sizes. There are syringes, dose cups, dose spoons, and nifty droppers. Your child will just need one for the dose that he commonly takes and is a size appropriate for his age. Beware that these measuring instruments will be labeled in the smallest print possible, with the oddest angles to read from, and most of the markings disappear off after the first washing. Count on it. Keep a few extras just in case.

If you have an infant or very small child who doesn't drink well from a cup, then plastic syringes and droppers are good choices. Syringes can also be used for the "premixed" doses for times when someone else is staying with the baby. You simply fill the syringe with the correct dosage, cap it, and use it when it's time for the next dose. Caution: remember to remove the little plastic cap before administering the medicine.

As your child gets older, she may not want the "baby" droppers, but may want to try medicine out of a dosing spoon. These are up-right spoons with a tube-like bottom. Once your child has a handle on holding and not spilling, a dose cup is in order. Measure the medicine while the cup is placed on a flat surface.

Deciding How Much to Administer

I have a big baby. She's just 16 months, but her weight is closer to that of a three year old. Should I give her medicine based on her weight or her age?

Thank goodness babies come in all shapes, sizes, and colors. Actually, weight-based dosing is much more accurate than age-based dosing and the daughter discussed above is a great example of why. In fact, doctors and hospitals routinely use the patient's weight to calculate the correct dosage. Often the calculations are done using a child's weight in kilograms. This isn't a difficult conversion; one kilogram equals 2.2 pounds. Here's an example. If a child weighs 22 pounds, that equals 11 kilograms. Twenty-two pounds in weight divided by 2.2 pounds equals 11 kilograms. Easy, right?

Very often, parents believe that just because a medicine is readily available over the counter, it will always be safe for children. Wrong! Read the labels carefully and check the dosage. Some manufacturers of off-the-shelf medicines get very tricky in terms of marketing. To have a greater percentage of the shelves filled with their products, they make many different formulations of the same product. For example, Tylenol does this type of marketing very well. Check the children's pain relief section carefully and you'll find a collection of suspensions, elixirs, concentrated drops, and chewable tablets, all with the same ingredient—acetaminophen—and all with the Tylenol name. The difference? The strength of the medicine in each dose.

A Drug Lady Recommendation

Take a "test drive" before you pour the medicine for real. Use plain water and try to approximate the correct dosage. Believe me, when you have a screaming child in one hand and a sticky medicine spoon in the other, you'll thank me.

In addition, use care when reading the doses on the label. I tell new parents to read the box, read the bottle, and then check it again just before you give the medicine. It's that serious.

Different strengths with the same medicine name sometimes get parents in trouble with the dosing for their child, especially if there are different ages of children in the home. For the suspension and elixir forms that older children take, the strength is 160mg in each teaspoonful. One teaspoonful is 5ml. However, for the concentrated Tylenol infant drops, the strength now changes to 160mg in 1.6ml or 500mg in one teaspoonful. Check dosages carefully before giving any medication to a child. When in doubt, ask a pediatrician or pharmacist.

Finding the Best-tasting Medicines

What is the best-tasting medicine for kids? We seem to have a constant battle getting medicine down. If there is a favorite flavor among small children, I'll be sure to get it next time!

"A spoonful of sugar helps the medicine go down?" Mary Poppins certainly had the right idea. Children's medicines now have all of the variety of a colorful candy store. Bubblegum and banana antibiotics, grape-flavored chewable pain relievers, and orange cough syrups are as common as chocolate and vanilla in the ice cream store. When a medicine has a really yucky taste, products have to go further to both mask the taste and make it taste like something appealing to youngsters.

As parents, this poses a challenge. You want your child to take a medicine when they are sick, but you don't want them to associate all medicines with candy. Balancing the line of caution and taking medicine is difficult with young children. It is never a good idea to refer to a medicine as candy, even if it means one dose will go down easier. If your back is turned just for a minute, the child could help himself to another "treat."

As with most everything else concerning children, the taste preferences of children can vary. Not only from child to child, but even from day to day! Thankfully, there are a few standards that most seem to like at one time or another. Cherry and grape are the old standbys; you'll see these flavors most often on the shelves.

There are pharmacies that will mix a specialty flavor for an especially disgusting medicine. The makers of the FLAVORx medicine flavoring system conducted a survey of a thousand parents nationwide and the results were quite startling. Ninety-six percent of parents said their children typically fail to take prescribed medicine as directed on the bottle. Eighty-five percent said that this failure to take the medicine caused the condition to last longer.

In places like children's clinics or hospitals where the little ones are given much smaller doses of adult medicines, taste is a big problem. When tablets must be crushed or harsh antibiotics given, adding a favorite flavor can make the difference in the medicine being taken or not.

If your child is too young to share what her favorite flavor is, then it's time to experiment. Cherry and grape flavors are first standards. Bubblegum and orange flavors are also great at masking the taste of medicine. If this doesn't work, try adding the medicine to a small amount of chocolate pudding, ice cream, or applesauce. Just be certain your child eats all of it to ensure the correct dosing. Most medicines can be safely mixed with these treats if it means the medicine will be taken. Check with a pharmacist if there is any uncertainty about a specific medicine. Inventiveness will have its own reward. If your child will take the medicine, then she will get better faster.

Dealing with Vague Box Instructions

My child is 16 months old. Previously, the doctor's office said to give Tylenol or Motrin for a fever. All of the over-the-counter products say for under the age of two consult a doctor. I called the doctor and no one will be in until Monday morning. What should I do?

As an accessible health care professional who just happens to be sitting beside the over-the-counter products, this is one of the most common questions I receive. It doesn't always make sense, but, for example, Infants' Tylenol Concentrated Drops do not provide an infant dosage on the box.

In a case like this, if a doctor has previously recommended use of Tylenol (acetaminophen) or Motrin (ibuprofen) for your child and you know their weight, the proper dose can be calculated by a pharmacist. Armed with a handy acetaminophen reference, the pharmacist will know that for a fever, the correct dosage is 15mg per kilogram of body weight. For ibuprofen, it's 10mg per kilogram of body weight. Remember, one kilogram equals 2.2 pounds. Also remember, there is quite a difference in strengths for common doses in concentrated infant drops, suspensions, elixirs, and chewable tablet forms. Common doses for both acetaminophen and ibuprofen are every four hours if needed, but it is necessary to read the instructions carefully for the particular product you purchased.

Guidelines for Safe Medication Use

We have four children from the ages of six months to nine years. One child has chronic asthma and one has ADHD that must be treated every day. With the combination of vitamins, cold medicines, and prescription medications, we could open a small pharmacy. How can I be sure that we are using all of these safely?

In a household as busy as the one above, it is extremely important to have certain guidelines for proper safe medication use and storage. It is also imperative to check and recheck dosages to ensure a child is receiving a safe and effective amount of medicine. Below are a few guidelines from the National Council on Patient Information and Education to tape to the inside of the medicine cabinet.

- If your child is taking more than one over-the-counter medicine, check the medicines for duplicate ingredients and usage.

- Don't give medicines in the dark. It's easy to make a mistake reading doses or product labels.

- Know your child's weight so you can measure the correct dose of medicine.

- Use the specific dropper, dosing cup, or other device that comes with your child's medicine. If it doesn't have one, ask a pharmacist for a calibrated measuring device.

■ Remember, babies and children should only take medications specifically formulated for their weight and age. Even a half or quarter of an adult dose may be an overdose for a child.

■ Teach children that medicines are not candy and they shouldn't touch, taste, or sniff them on their own. Keep all medicines, including vitamins, out of children's reach.

■ Follow label directions carefully.

■ If ever in doubt about which medicine to give your child or how to give it correctly, ask a doctor or pharmacist.

■ Talk with a doctor about other medicines your child is taking, including over-the-counter products, before the doctor writes a prescription.

The Fluoride Supplementation
Controversy

The school nurse asked if my children were taking fluoride supplements. I asked if they should be and she didn't know. The doctor's office said they would prescribe some for the children if I wanted it. Do I want fluoride for my child?

This is a dilemma shared by many parents. The debate over whether to add fluoride supplements to your child's daily regimen depends on several factors:

- Where you and your child live.

- How much fluoride is in the water supply.

- How much fluoride your child may be getting from other sources—for example their formula or school water.

Over 30 percent of the population lives in an area without public water fluoridation. If you live in one of those places and have a private well or a community system that does not add fluoride to the water, you'll have to decide whether or not to provide flouride supplements to your child. Ask a dentist or public water company what the local water fluoride level is.

Fluoride concentration is measured in parts per million (ppm). If the water in your area has one part fluoride per one million parts water (1ppm), this will prevent tooth decay in 60 percent of children. A glass of 1ppm water is equal to a 0.25mg flouride tablet. The concentrations of fluoride can also vary from area to area. The United States Public Health Service established the optimum concentration for fluoride in the water in the United States in the range of 0.7 to 1.2 ppm.

Following are the American Dental Association (ADA) guidelines for additional fluoride supplementation based on your child's age and the amount of fluoridation in your water.

Age	Fluoride ion level in drinking water (ppm)		
	<0.3ppm	0.3–0.6 ppm	>0.6 ppm
Birth–6 months	None	None	None
6 months–3 years	0.25mg/day	None	None
3–6 years	0.50mg/day	0.25mg/day	None
6–16 years	1.0mg/day	0.50mg/day	None

Another aspect of the fluoride debate is whether or not adding fluoride to the public water supply is the responsibility of government agencies. Some individuals see fluoridation of public water as limiting their freedom of choice. Others have concerns of increased cancer risks or increased risk of toxicity from an element placed in something as difficult to control as a municipal water supply.

Looking at the studies as a health care provider, I have found no cause for undue concern about the safety of our water supplies in regard to fluoride treatment and overwhelming evidence that fluoridation prevents tooth decay. Adding fluoride to the water simply provides an individual with an increased level of protection against developing dental disease. Water that has been fortified with fluoride has no more risks than those of adding vitamin C to orange juice and vitamin D to milk.

Fluoride Benefits

To help you decide, here are a few facts about fluoride that you might want to know. First, fluoride is the most effective agent available to prevent tooth decay. The National Institutes of Health recommend fluoride supplementation as safe, inexpensive, and effective for tooth decay prevention.

A study cited in the *Journal of Public Health* showed that school-aged children who lived all of their lives in a community with good water fluoride levels had a 61 to 100 percent less incidence of tooth decay than children who had low fluoride levels in their drinking water. Another study found that children in lower socioeconomic groups also derive benefits from water fluoridation with an average 54 percent reduction in tooth decay.

Fluoride protects teeth that you can see, as well as those still invisible and growing below the gum line. It is thought to work by binding to developing teeth and forming a barrier, called a fluoride hydroxyapatite, that prevents tooth-damaging bacteria and plaque from sticking to the surface.

According the ADA, fluoride has a positive effect in two ways: the availability of topical fluoride in the mouth during the initial formation of decay can not only stop the decay process, but also make the enamel surface more resistant to future acid attacks. Additionally, the presence of fluoride in saliva provides a reservoir of fluoride ions that can be incorporated into the tooth surface to prevent decay.

For children not getting enough fluoride, there are obvious signs. Teeth may be unsightly from decay, more teeth may be lost due to root cavities, and the child may spend more time visiting the dentist for fillings. Dental bills must be put into the family budget or the child can suffer problems with self-esteem, and possibly develop problems chewing or speaking correctly.

Fluoride Dangers

The danger of too much fluoride is a condition called dental fluorosis. When there is more fluoride available than the developing tooth can safely absorb, white spots appear on the tooth surface. The spots appear as patchy areas, and in severe cases, as brown stains.

With dental fluorosis, there is a narrow window of time for damage to occur. The child's permanent teeth begin to form enamel from about the time of birth until approximately five years of age. After tooth enamel is completely formed, dental fluorosis cannot develop even if higher levels of fluoride are ingested.

In order to decrease the risk of dental fluorosis in permanent teeth, fluoride supplements should only be prescribed for children living in nonfluoridated areas. The correct amount of a fluoride supplement is based on the child's age and the existing fluoride level in the drinking water.

Fluoride may also be present in foods your child eats every day. Although the concentration of fluoride depends on how much fluoride was present in the water and soil, foods like apples and eggs may contain high levels of fluoride.

Some schools have their own fluoridation systems in place. Here a much larger concentration of fluoride (up to four-and-one-half times

A Drug Lady Reminder

Children under the age of six should be closely watched when they are using a fluoride toothpaste. It's easy for them to gob large amounts on the toothbrush from unwieldy tubes. Just a pea-sized dab of toothpaste should be put on their toothbrushes to avoid excess fluoride.

Oragel Toddler Training Toothpaste is a fluoride-free way to teach good brushing habits without adding excess abrasives or foaming action.

the amount in public water supplies) is used to compensate for the time children are not in school. Check with your child's school to find out if there is such a program in place.

Fluoride toxicity, as in an accidental overdose of a fluoride-containing product, can be life-threatening. The symptoms include stomach pain, excessive drooling, nausea, vomiting, excessive thirst, tremors, and diarrhea.

Products Available

FLUORIDE TOOTHPASTE

Using a toothpaste and toothbrush can effectively put fluoride directly on the surface of, and partially in between, the teeth. For children living in areas with no fluoridation, brushing alone may not be enough to completely protect the teeth.

RINSES AND GELS

Studies have shown that for children living in areas with nonfluoridated water, washing the mouth with a 0.05 percent sodium fluoride rinse resulted in a significant reduction in cavities. These rinses are also a good choice for teens with braces. Because of the difficulty of brushing around the orthodontics, a rinse provides good protection.

Children aged six to 12 should be supervised closely while using these products to ensure they are following label directions to the letter and rinsing the mouth properly after use. Consult with a dentist or pediatrician for those under six, as they may swallow more than is safe.

Here are some guidelines for using topical (in the mouth) fluoride treatments:

■ Carefully measure the dose on the package and apply to the teeth for one minute (if liquid, swish vigorously).

■ Use no more than once a day.

■ When finished, spit out the product completely. Don't swallow it.

■ Rinse mouth thoroughly with water.

■ Don't eat or drink for 30 minutes after treatment.

PRESCRIPTION SUPPLEMENTS

For children who do not live in fluoridated communities, prescription fluoride supplements are an effective alternative to water fluoridation for the prevention of tooth decay. The general recommendation is to add supplements in areas where water fluoride concentrations are less than 0.3ppm. Fluoride supplements are available in two forms: liquid drops for infants aged six months and up, and chewable tablets for children and adolescents.

For children from six months to the age that they can chew tablets, liquid fluoride supplements like Luride (sodium fluoride) can be prescribed. For those aged six months to three years, the dose is 0.25mg (or a half dropperful) daily. There is also a combination fluoride product with a liquid multivitamin called Poly-Vi-Flor.

Chewable sodium fluoride tablets come in 1.1mg and 2.2mg doses and in a variety of flavors. For children aged three to six years, the dose is 1.1mg (this equals .5mg of actual fluoride). For those six to twelve years, the daily dose is a 2.2mg tablet (equivalent to 1mg of actual fluoride). While these may taste good to your child, always keep them away from little hands to prevent an accidental overdose.

Fluoride supplement dosing should be only once a day and spaced apart from milk or dairy products by at least an hour. Two hours is even better. These products can decrease the amount of fluoride absorbed into the child's system.

What the Experts Say

The National Institute of Dental Research claims, "The use of a fluoride-containing dentifrice (toothpaste) is recommended for children and adults. Regular and thorough brushing with a fluoride dentifrice will provide protection against tooth decay and added protection when used together with most other forms of fluoride therapy."

Food Allergies

Food allergies in children can be a truly frightening experience. A child may take a bite of something they may have eaten before without incident, then suddenly begin to itch and turn red. The throat may swell, making it difficult to breathe. If not attended to quickly, the child may go into shock and die. After ensuring a child receives prompt medical treatment, parents must begin the vigilant process of trying to guarantee that the child never is exposed to that particular food again.

Children with parents who have allergies or asthma are at much greater risk for developing food allergies. In the United States, there are approximately 29,000 food-related anaphylactic reactions (see Anaphylactic Shock, pg. 138) each year, and a small percentage of these are fatal. In most cases, the individual was not aware they had consumed a forbidden food. Reading ingredient labels for all foods is the key to maintaining control over the allergy. If a product doesn't have a label, those with allergies should not eat that food. If a label contains an unfamiliar term, parents must call the manufacturer and ask for a definition of that term or avoid allowing a child to eat that food.

Food allergies strike six to eight percent of children, especially infants and those under the age of two. The good news is that with some food allergies, like those to milk, the majority of children will grow out of them. The bad news is that most allergies to peanuts or tree nuts are life-long. Strict avoidance of the allergy-causing food is the only way to avoid a reaction. The most common foods causing allergic reactions are peanuts, soy, wheat, shellfish, fish, milk, eggs, and tree nuts.

Allergies vs. Food Sensitivities

While only six to eight percent of children have true food allergies, studies show that parents perceive that a food allergy is present in over 20 percent of children. There are different types of food reactions. True food allergies require immediate medical treatment. Food sensitivities, while not pleasant, typically can be controlled with home care and vigilance.

During the early years, a child may become sensitized to a particular food protein, like those in eggs or peanuts. For the first several times the food is eaten, there is no unusual reaction noticed. However, the child's immune system is developing antibodies against the protein. The next time the child eats the offending food, the body reacts to it as though it is a foreign substance that must be removed at all costs. The cells release large amounts of histamine into the blood, triggering an anaphylactic response.

Allergic reactions to foods are divided into several categories:

■ **Immediate (type I) hypersensitivity.** When an immediate Type I food reaction occurs, the child experiences symptoms within five to 30 minutes of having ingested the food. Symptom onset is rapid and may include tingling of the extremities, facial swelling, itching, wheezing, coughing, vomiting, flushing of the skin, tightening of the throat, nausea, abdominal cramps, and diarrhea. Sometimes in cases where nuts, shellfish, fish, and peanuts have been eaten, anaphylactic shock can occur.

■ **Oral allergy syndrome.** Oral allergy syndrome occurs when the child eats certain fresh fruits, like strawberries, melons, kiwi, or certain fresh vegetables, like celery or carrots. The lips and tongue become swollen and red, and the child may have intense itching around the mouth area. This type of allergy typically gets better with the use of antihistamines (like diphenhydramine).

■ **Respiratory hypersensitivity.** This occurs when a child is exposed to fumes or smells from a food to which he is allergic. The symptoms are sneezing, runny nose, congestion, wheezing, or coughing. A child with this form of food allergy typically needs daily asthma control medication.

■ **Delayed food allergy.** A delayed food allergy can take up to three days to appear. Unlike an immediate food reaction, delayed food reaction is not a fixed food allergy. For example, if a child were allergic to milk and increased his intake and/or frequency of milk consumption, it would be after the increase that symptoms would likely appear. This type of allergy is identified by the IgG antibodies present (rather than IgE antibodies of the immediate reactions).

■ **Food sensitivity.** A food intolerance or sensitivity is an adverse food-induced reaction that does not involve the immune system. Lactose intolerance is one example of a food intolerance. A person with lactose intolerance lacks an enzyme that is needed to digest milk sugar. When the child eats milk products, symptoms such as gas, bloating, and abdominal pain may occur.

Diagnosing Food Allergies

If your child experiences all the symptoms of a food allergy, it may not always be easy to identify the cause of the reaction. In such a case, your child's doctor will try to identify the specific antigens present. The skin prick test (SPT) is usually done first. The SPT involves placing a drop of extract from the suspected food culprit on the patient's forearm or back and pricking the skin. If the patient is allergic to the food, a red, raised bump (like a mosquito bite) will appear on the site. If the SPT result is negative, there is 90 percent chance the child is not allergic to that food. Unfortunately, a positive SPT to a food is only about 50 percent accurate.

Therefore, if there is a positive result, the doctor will also order a radioallergosorbent (RAST) or ImmunoCAP FEIA (fluoroenzyme immunoassay) blood test, which can confirm the IgE-mediated allergies that tested positive on the SPT. If the results are still inconclusive, the child's doctor may request that a diet diary be completed. This diary is a detailed chronological record of all the foods the child ate, or simply put in his mouth, over a specific period. Once the diary is completed, there is typically a four- to six-week trial; the health care provider, child, and parents will review it to identify connections between the child's food and symptoms. An elimination diet may also be ordered to identify the source of a reaction. With this diet, the child must cut out those foods suspected of causing a reaction. His family and health care team will then monitor him for reactions.

If blood tests, a diet diary, and an elimination diet do not pinpoint a clear relationship between a specific food and a child's symptoms, a food challenge may be ordered. In a food challenge, the patient eats the suspected foods in gradually increasing quantities in a controlled and monitored setting, under the close supervision of an allergist. The choice of foods to be tested is based upon the patient's history plus skin and blood test results.

Reading Labels

A distinct problem that has been identified recently is the inability of current food ingredient labels to easily provide vital information to parents with food-allergic children. Parents of severely allergic children were asked to review labels from many commercially available products and the results were disturbing. Only seven percent were able to identify milk listed under different names or product ingredients. Only 54 percent were able to identify all products containing peanuts, with 22 percent correctly identifying soy or soy protein products.

Parents must realize that ingredients can change without a warning appearing on the front of the product, so reading the label is a requirement with every shopping trip. Any questions or concerns have to be addressed to the manufacturer, asking if the product contains milk or peanuts or whatever ingredient your child is allergic to.

The Food Allergy & Anaphylaxis Network (FAAN), available at www.faan.org, provides a laminated, wallet-sized card to train parents of food-allergic children how to identify common food allergens on labels.

Hidden Dangers

Scouring food labels to locate potentially harmful ingredients for your child can be a daunting experience. To make matters worse, ingredient labels may use different names for the same product. Here are some allergy-producing foods and the "other" names they may go by on an ingredients label:

■ Eggs: Albumin, globulin, livetin, ovalbumin (and other products beginning with "ov"), powdered egg, silici albuminate, vitellin yolk, dried egg

■ Fish: Surimi (imitation crabmeat), shrimp, and shellfish

■ Milk: Casein (a milk derivative), sodium caseinate, whey, ghee, lactalbumin, lactoferrin

■ Peanuts: Mandelonas (peanuts soaked in almond flavoring), arachis oil, peanut oil

■ Soy: Soya, hydrologized protein, lecithin, textured vegetable protein

■ Tree nuts: Artificial nuts, which can be peanuts reflavored as another type of nut, such as a pecan or walnut

■ Wheat: Spelt, gluten, cereal extract, couscous, durum, seminola

Other hidden food allergy dangers can occur when an allergenic food is found in prepared foods. Here are some examples:

■ Eggs: Found in mayonnaise, meringues, egg substitutes, surimi, fat substitutes such as Simplesse, egg noodles, baked goods, root beer, some cake icing, and foam or milky toppings on specialty coffee drinks

■ Fish, shellfish: Found in caponata (a relish of chopped eggplant), Caesar salad dressings, and Worcestershire sauces, which often contain anchovies. Hot dogs, bologna, and pizza toppings may contain surimi.

■ Milk: Found in some margarines, processed meats such as hot dogs and bologna, canned fish, coffee whiteners, candy, instant breakfast drinks, caramel food coloring and flavoring, and fat substitutes

■ Peanuts: Found in peanut butter, peanut oil, peanut flour, M&Ms (plain and with nuts), jelly beans, chocolate, candy bars, pastries, pie crusts, egg rolls, and other Chinese dishes, as well as Mexican, Thai, and Vietnamese food

■ Soy: Found in soy, teriyaki, and Worcestershire sauces; tofu; miso; baked goods using soy flour or oil; soy nuts; infant formulas; sauces; soups; soybean paste; tuna packed in vegetable oil; and many margarines

■ Tree nuts (walnuts, cashews): Found in barbecue sauce, cereal, crackers, ice cream, pastries, chocolate, suntan lotion, and shampoo

■ Wheat: Found in most baked goods, many processed meats, gravy, pasta, some canned soups, distilled vinegar, and modified food starch

Everyday Life with Food Allergies

When everything that touches your child's lips must be monitored to prevent a potentially life-threatening incident, a parent's responsibility becomes enormous. Because strict avoidance is the only treatment for a food allergy, the family must make many changes to things they might have taken for granted before.

The family must also be prepared to face the very real chance that the child will come into contact with the food allergen again. This happens in over 60 percent of the cases of food allergies discovered, and most of the time, the child was unaware they had consumed something forbidden.

The first step is to ensure that medication is available. The EpiPen (epinephrine) is available by doctor's prescription. It is important to have several around the home, in the diaper bag or backpack, and at school. Your child's doctor or pharmacist can train you how to use the EpiPen properly *before* a reaction occurs. Remember that prompt medical attention is always required after an EpiPen is used, as it only contains a small amount of potentially life-saving medicine.

It is necessary for all family members to periodically review a written Food Allergy Action plan. Forms for these plans can be downloaded from FAAN (www.faan.org). Included are instructions for administering the EpiPen and important numbers to call during a reaction. These forms should also be distributed to your child's extended family, teachers, day care workers, and coaches.

SCHOOL

There are approximately two million schoolchildren who suffer from food allergies, so many school officials are familiar with caring for these children. Schools are required to administer the child's EpiPen during a reaction, even if no school nurse is available. This is when the Food Allergy Action plan becomes important.

Many parents provide "safe" foods for their child to eat at school and more schools are promoting a "no food trading" policy to reduce the chance the child might encounter an allergenic food.

FAMILY

Parents of a food-allergic child may choose to provide safe foods for the entire family, so the allergic child doesn't feel isolated. Others choose to teach the child about which food to avoid and set up designated areas where "safe" and "unsafe" foods are kept and prepared.

All meals for an allergic child should be cooked separately from the rest of the family's food. It should first be prepared, then covered and removed from the cooking area to prevent contamination by the unsafe foods.

RESTAURANTS

Parents of an allergic child should speak to the restaurant manager about the child's allergies and ask about the ingredients in the foods the child wishes to eat. Even foods as simple as French fries could be fried in the same oils as fish (triggering an allergy to fish), use peanut oil (triggering a peanut allergy), or have crumbs from another food breaded with wheat flour (triggering a wheat allergy).

Families with a food-allergic child must make conscious and careful decisions regarding food choices in a restaurant setting. Hidden allergy dangers lurk in sauces, desserts, and even utensils that could become contaminated if used to prepare other foods.

8

HIV/AIDS in Children

The Definition of HIV/AIDS

HIV (the human immunodeficiency virus) attacks and gradually weakens the immune system by destroying the CD4+ cells, a type of white blood cell. White blood cells are an important part of the immune system, which helps a child fight infections. HIV contributes to AIDS (acquired immunodeficiency syndrome). However, a child with the HIV virus may not have AIDS. AIDS is diagnosed once a child's immune system is weakened to the point where certain types of life-threatening diseases, infections, and cancers can take hold. AIDS is the most advanced stage of HIV infection.

The Diagnosis of HIV

Infants and young children infected with HIV often show "failure to thrive" symptoms. This means that the child doesn't grow, gain weight, or mature developmentally at the same rate as healthy children. A DNA test, called a PCR (polymerase chain reaction), can determine if a child simply has antibodies to HIV from her mother or if she actually has the infection herself. This test now allows diagnosis by 14 to 30 days of life in most children. Two positive blood tests drawn at two separate times are considered diagnostic of HIV infection. Children with HIV may also have frequent or chronic diarrhea, frequent minor bacterial infections such as otitis media and sinusitis, and thrush. Extensive warts or noninfectious skin manifestations such as rashes should raise the suspicion of HIV infection.

Statistics

Worldwide, approximately 25 million people have died of AIDS since the beginning of the epidemic, thought to have begun in the late 1970s, approximately five million of them being children. In 2003, three million people died of AIDS; 500,000 (1,600 per day) of them were children. Mother-to-child transmission of HIV through perinatal infection has accounted for 91 percent of all AIDS cases reported among U.S. children. Of children born to HIV-infected mothers, 20 to 40 percent will be infected themselves. In the case of those infected from their mothers, as many as 50 percent will die before their second birthday.

During the reporting period from 1999 until December 2002 the highest incidence of AIDS in women in the United States occurs in the District of Columbia, New York, Florida, Maryland, Puerto Rico, and the Virgin Islands. The greatest rate of increase, however, has been in the South. The greatest numbers of infected children live in New York, Florida, New Jersey, Texas, and California. HIV-infected women and children in the United States are disproportionately black or Hispanic. More than 80 percent of children diagnosed with AIDS in the most recent reporting period were black or Hispanic.

Complications

OPPORTUNISTIC INFECTIONS

HIV-infected infants and children will be more prone to ordinary infections, like colds and earaches. Chronic diarrhea and thrush, caused by the yeast *Candida,* are also frequent (see Diarrhea, pg. 201).

Children with a compromised immune system are much more susceptible to opportunistic infections (OIs). OIs can occur quickly in HIV children and can be deadly. The child has no antibodies to fight the typical infections that children are exposed to. Serious bacterial and viral infections, like pneumocystis carinii pneumonia (PCP), lympocytic interstial pneumonitis (LIP), and cytomegalovirus (CMV), are especially dangerous for HIV children.

MALNUTRITION

Malnutrition is a common complication of HIV infection and AIDS. Malnutrition places added stress on an already weakened immune system and may complicate the treatment of the disease by affecting the intestinal tract's ability to absorb drugs, as well as its ability to absorb proteins, carbohydrates, and fats. Malnutrition in children is particularly devastating because children are still growing and developing, placing even higher energy demands on their bodies and immune systems. All children, regardless of the stage of their infection, should be seen by a registered dietitian (RD) for a thorough assessment and evaluation. It has been estimated that over 90 percent of children with HIV infection/AIDS will experience delayed growth. The reasons for this are poor socioeconomic situations, poor nutritional intake, the inability of the body to absorb food, and the disease itself.

A frequently used and tolerated intervention is to encourage small, frequent feedings instead of a traditional three-meal pattern. Parents and caregivers may feel that unless the child is eating three meals they are not getting adequate nutrition. It is important to remember if several smaller meals and snacks are given instead of the traditional three that these are planned appropriately in regard to the child's medication schedule.

Sufficient calories and protein can be provided with supplements. Formulas can be boosted with medical nutritionals such as carbohydrate sources (Polycose), protein sources (Promod, Meritene), or fat sources (Microlipid). Other supplements available for older children—those one to ten years of age—include Pediasure, Instant Breakfast–type drinks, Resource, and Scandishake. These are available at your pharmacy or grocery store. It is also recommended that vitamin and mineral supplements be given for all children, regardless of the stage of infection. One that provides 100 percent of the recommended daily allowance for the age range of the child is appropriate. For older children and adolescents, an adult vitamin is appropriate.

VACCINATIONS

There are a few recommendations regarding HIV-infected children that differ from those for HIV-negative children. Encapsulated bacteria cause considerable problems for HIV-infected children, so *Haemophilus influenzae* and pneumonia vaccines are important. Chicken pox (varicella) vaccine is a live virus vaccine, but it can be considered for HIV-infected children without immunosuppression. Measles, mumps, and rubella vaccine can be safely given to HIV-infected children who do not have severe immunosuppression (considered a Category 3 disease).

Children's Medications

Ideally, prenatal HIV testing will identify those infants at risk for HIV due to an infected mother. Use of antiretroviral medications during pregnancy and delivery will prevent HIV transmission in up to 99 percent of cases. For those children born to HIV-infected mothers, zidovudine will be administered every six hours beginning within a few hours of birth, and will continue for four to six weeks.

A combination regimen with three drugs is the preferred follow-up. Clinical trials showed evidence of clinical benefit and/or sustained suppression of HIV replication in children who underwent this regimen. This is strongly recommended as first-line therapy. The two alternative regimens are:

■ One highly active protease inhibitor plus two nucleoside analogue reverse transcriptase inhibitors (NRTIs). The preferred protease inhibitor for infants and children who cannot swallow pills or capsules is nelfinavir or ritonavir. For those children who can swallow pills or capsules, indinavir is preferred.

■ Recommended dual. Most data on use in children recommends the combinations of zidovudine and didanosine and zidovudine and lamivudine for the NRTI combination.

■ For those children who can swallow capsules, efavirenz (Sustiva) plus two NRTIs, as above, or efavirenz (Sustiva) plus nelfinavir and one NRTI, as above.

Once initiated, antiretroviral therapy will likely be life-long. The greatest body of data in children is from studies using two NRTIs and a protease inhibitor. Nelfinavir (Viracept) and ritonavir (Norvir) are available in pediatric formulations and are preferred for children too young to swallow pills. Nelfinavir is available as a powder, but crushed tablets are generally better tolerated and get into the system more rapidly. For children who can swallow capsules, indinavir (Crixivan) or saquinavir soft-gel capsules (Fortovase) may be used.

Young children, especially those under six, have a great advantage over older children in terms of their ability to beat the disease. Their immune systems are able to regenerate cells at a faster rate, and in many cases, return to normal levels after treatment, in a process called seroreversion.

Taking Care of the HIV Child

In home settings, it is important to use precautions to prevent the rare spread of the disease to the caregiver or other family members. Here are some tips:

■ Wear gloves during contact with blood or other body fluids that could possibly contain visible blood, such as urine, feces, or vomit.

■ Cover cuts, sores, or breaks in the skin with bandages (this goes for the caregivers as well as the infected child).

■ Wash hands (or any body part touched) immediately after contact with blood or other body fluids.

■ Avoid sharing toothbrushes.

■ Dispose of used needles in "sharps" containers available from the pharmacy.

The care of children with HIV is a complex undertaking. Ideally, a comprehensive care team should be available, including a physician, nurse, pharmacist, social worker, nutritionist, and mental health professional.

Once a team is in place, it is important that all members are kept informed about the child's condition. It is important to ask questions about a child's condition, medications, progress, or anything that is confusing.

Learn the names of a child's medicines and possible side effects. If the child misses a dose or takes half the dose, or if they stop early, the virus or bacteria can learn to survive the medicine. Sometimes this causes it to change or get stronger. Then the medicine no longer works. This is called resistance. This is a very big worry for doctors, nurses, and pharmacists who treat children with HIV infection. It is a big worry for people living with HIV. (see the Dangers of Antibiotic Resistance, page 29). Following are some tips from the Elizabeth Glaser Pediatric AIDS Foundation (www.pedaids.org) to make giving and taking medications easier:

- Make a schedule for medicines and daily eating times that will work for the caregiver and the child. The nurse, pharmacist, or doctor can help with fitting the medicines into this schedule.

- Use reminders. Use a calendar or check-off list. Tape the calendar someplace visible. The front of the refrigerator is a good place. Check off each dose that is given to the child.

- Use timers or a watch with an alarm as a reminder to give the dose.

- Color-code the bottles of liquid medicines with matching oral syringes. This helps make giving the right dose easier. Put the same color for the medicine on the calendar or checklist.

■ Use a special dosing cup, measuring spoon, or an oral syringe to measure the right amount of the medicine. Don't use eating spoons to measure liquid medicines as their size may vary.

■ Pack the drugs in one-week packets and check weekly that all doses are given.

HIV infection entails special psychosocial problems for children. The diagnosis carries with it the fear of rejection and the inability to feel "normal." Repeated medical visits, procedures, and complicated medical regimens are stressful and can make the child feel different and isolated. Most of all encourage the child to do things other children do. Let her play and have friends. Let her be a normal child.

9

Insect Repellants

To spray or not to spray?

Many parents worry that covering their child in a product that causes violent death to an insect could not be safe for the child. In fact, insect repellant sprays or lotions for human use don't actually kill the bugs, but repel them and encourage them to find another body to bite.

Commercial products are available in many forms, including those with DEET, citronella, soybean oil, and bath oil as their active ingredients. Devices, like the Mosquito Deleto and Mosquito Magnet, attempt to lure mosquitoes away from the family and trap them safely in a container.

Why a Bug Bites

Bugs bite either to eat (mosquitoes, biting gnats, ticks, fleas) or to protect themselves from perceived danger (bees, wasps, fire ants). Female mosquitoes bite people and animals because they need the protein found in blood to help develop their eggs.

Insect repellants won't protect against those biting insects that respond to danger. Mosquitoes and other insects that use a child as a food source respond differently. The mosquito follows the trail of carbon dioxide that a child breathes out. The insect is also attracted to the warmth, sweat chemicals, and carbon dioxide that the skin emits. The insect will begin a zigzag course until it locates the child. Insect repellant works by masking these signals, fooling the insect and convincing it that something else would be a better lunch.

The best prevention against these pests is to avoid the bite entirely. Here are some ways to help your child avoid getting a bite:

- Have your child wear long-sleeved shirts and long pants wherever biting insects congregate.

- Have your child wear light-colored clothing, as dark colors and heat often attract insects.

- Avoid heavily scented lotions, soaps, and shampoos on your child, as these can make it easier for insects to find him.

- Have your child avoid areas with insect nests or where insects appear to swarm.

The Dangers of Insect Repellants

Because a very young child's skin can absorb chemicals readily, parents should be careful when using commercial insect repellants on this age group.

- Apply insect repellants to clothing instead of the skin to reduce the amount absorbed.

■ Don't apply near the eyes, mouth, open cuts, or scrapes, or on the hands of small children.

■ Wash off insect repellants as soon as the bug danger is over.

■ Follow the instructions carefully on the bottle of the insect repellant used.

■ Don't allow children to handle insect repellants or put it on themselves.

■ Don't use insect repellants near food and avoid spraying in enclosed areas (like tents) to prevent the child from breathing the vapors.

DEET

DEET (N, N-diethyl-3-methylbenzamide) is the only mosquito repellant the Centers for Disease Control (CDC) recommends for preventing mosquito-borne diseases. It's been around since 1946 and is still the most effective for bite avoidance. Some parents still associate DEET with the now banned insecticide DDT, even though these are entirely different products.

According to the American Academy of Pediatrics (AAP), products containing DEET are very safe when used according to the directions. Because DEET is so widely used, a great deal of testing has been done. Parents should always supervise or put DEET-containing insect repellants on young children themselves, but the AAP has given the green light for DEET use on children as young as two months old and has raised the maximum DEET concentration in mosquito repellant for kids from ten to 30 percent.

Children can and should use both sunscreen and DEET when they are outdoors to protect their health. Follow the instructions on the package for proper application of each product. Apply sunscreen first, followed by repellant containing DEET.

The percentage of DEET in a product determines the amount of protection your child will receive. One recent study showed:

■ A product containing 23.8 percent DEET provided an average of five hours of protection from mosquito bites.

■ A product containing 20 percent DEET provided almost four hours of protection.

■ A product with 6.65 percent DEET provided almost two hours of protection.

■ Products with 4.75 percent DEET and two percent soybean oil were able to provide roughly one-and-a-half hours of protection.

If you have concerns about the safety of DEET, the National Pesticide Information Center (NPIC) has the latest information about active ingredients and possible dangers of insect repellants. NPIC is available at 1-800-858-7378 or www.npic.orst.edu.

Products

Insect repellants can be found in many different forms and concentrations. Sprays, lotions, sticks, and creams are available for direct skin application, and some aerosols are meant for direct on-the-clothes applications. The Environmental Protection Agency (EPA) recommends checking the product container to ensure that it has an EPA-approved label and registration number. Follow directions carefully and store the products out of children's reach. Use just enough to cover exposed skin and clothing.

Following are a few EPA-approved and -tested products:

■ **OFF Skintastic Magicolor Disappearing Purple.** Kids like this one because it coats the skin in a purple color to let the child know that he's covered completely, then disappears. It repels gnats, mosquitoes, biting flies, fleas, ticks, and no-see-ums.

■ **OFF! Deep Woods.** This product contains 24 percent DEET and gave the best protection, according to a 2002 *New England Journal of Medicine* study. The protection lasted a full five hours.

■ **Avon Skin-So-Soft Bug Guard Plus.** This protects against mosquitoes, deer ticks, black flies, gnats, and no-see-ums. It is hypoallergenic, DEET free, and PABA free.

■ **OFF Botanicals Plant-Based Insect Repellant.** This uses eucalyptus-based ingredients. It repels mosquitoes, black flies, gnats, and no-see-ums.

Spray Alternatives

SKIN-SO-SOFT
This bath oil product has been used for many years as an effective insect repellant. However, studies show that this product doesn't offer the same level of protection, or that protection does not last as long as products containing DEET.

CATNIP OIL
According to an Iowa State University study, the essential oil of catnip proved up to ten times more potent than DEET in fending off mos-

quitoes. The tests were done using the oil on clothing and not on the skin, but more products containing this oil will likely be produced in the future.

MOSQUITO DELETO AND MOSQUITO MAGNET

These portable devices emit a steady stream of carbon dioxide, along with the chemical octenol. Placing these devices away from people lures mosquitoes into the traps where they collect and die. Studies show that these products trap huge numbers of mosquitoes in a short period of time, but whether they reduce bites from mosquitoes already present is not yet known.

BUG ZAPPERS

Bug zappers emit florescent light to attract bugs where they are loudly and effectively terminated. Unfortunately, mosquitoes and most biting insects aren't attracted to florescent light. Bug zappers also kill many beneficial insects that don't mean any harm to a child.

WRIST BANDS

Wrist bands impregnated with DEET or citronella are certainly convenient, but there is little evidence to support that they work to repel biting insects. Because the insect repellant needs to be applied to the skin to mask the mosquito-attracting chemicals, studies show that biting insects had no problem biting the skin within inches of the wrist band.

West Nile Virus

DEFINITION

This mosquito-borne virus is definitely something to take seriously. West Nile virus has killed nearly 300 people in the United States since

1999. The vast majority of people (99 percent) bitten by a mosquito infected with West Nile don't know they have the disease. However, for those that do develop the disease, a paralyzing polio-like condition or even death may occur. Other survivors of serious West Nile virus infection may have permanent nerve damage or long-lasting fatigue.

THE SYMPTOMS OF WEST NILE VIRUS

The time from infection to the first sign of symptoms of the West Nile virus is usually three to 14 days. Most infections are mild, and symptoms include fever, headache, body aches (flu-like symptoms), and occasionally a skin rash and swollen lymph nodes. Infections that are more serious may cause encephalitis, which is a swelling and inflammation of the brain. The following other symptoms may also be present:

- Headache
- High fever
- Stiff neck
- Disorientation
- Reduced attention to surroundings
- Tremors and convulsions
- Muscle weakness or paralysis
- Coma

If you suspect that your child may have contracted the West Nile virus, it is important to contact the doctor immediately. While there is no medication to cure West Nile infection, supportive treatment for the virus includes intravenous fluids and respiratory support on a ventilator if needed.

HOW TO AVOID WEST NILE VIRUS

Many of the mosquitoes that carry the West Nile virus are especially likely to bite around dusk and dawn. If the family is outdoors around these times of the day, it is important to apply repellant to your child. In other parts of the country, there are mosquitoes that also bite during the day, and these mosquitoes have also been found to carry the West Nile virus. The safest decision is to apply mosquito repellant whenever you are outdoors.

Avoid areas where mosquitoes may congregate and lay their eggs, like garbage cans, stagnant pools of water, or wet, wooded areas.

Officials in the area may use fogger sprays with airborn insecticides that kill mosquitoes, to blanket cities most at risk for West Nile virus. The CDC carefully examines the amount of chemicals used to ensure that there are only enough to kill the mosquito population. The CDC also periodically tests those exposed to the mosquito fog to guarantee blood levels of the pesticide remain at safe levels. It is still important to use a mosquito repellant whenever there is risk of contact with the insects.

Lyme Disease and
Rocky Mountain Spotted Fever

DANGERS

Lyme disease (see Lyme Disease, pg. 265) is the leading tick-borne disease in the United States. Rocky Mountain spotted fever is another concern in high tick infestation areas. Ticks are most active from April through October, so it is important to use special care when your child is outdoors during those times. Any insect repellant chosen for your child should clearly state that it effectively repels ticks, as not all do.

AVOIDING INFECTION

The best way to avoid infection from a tick is to avoid the bite entirely. To keep ticks away, dress your child in long-sleeved shirts and long pants, with the pants cuffs tucked into her socks or boots. Light-colored clothing will reveal ticks before they have a chance to find a home. It is also important to inspect your child carefully after forays into the forest or high grass. If you find a tick on your child, remove it carefully and contact the doctor for further instructions.

REMOVING TICKS

To remove a tick on your child:

■ Use fine-point tweezers to grasp the tick as close to the skin as possible.

■ Pull gently. Avoid squeezing the body of the tick.

■ Clean the site of the bite, your hands, and the tweezers with disinfectant.

■ Consider wearing protective gloves.

You also may want to place the tick in a small container, like a pill container, and bring it to your doctor, pharmacist, or veterinarian for identification. Never use a burned match, petroleum jelly, or nail polish to try to remove ticks. These methods are ineffective.

Overweight Children:
A New Health Crisis

The number of children defined as overweight (at or above the ninety-fifth percentile of Body Mass Index for their age and gender) has doubled in the last 20 years. The rate of overweight boys has quadrupled in the last 25 years. Ten percent of preschoolers (between the ages of two and five) are overweight, up from seven percent in 1994. Current figures put the total number of overweight children between the ages of six and 19 at just over nine million! Obesity has become one of the fastest growing epidemics for American children today.

Reasons for this increase in weight for the younger set appear to be a lack of activity and poor eating habits. These same problems can be seen in the adult population as well. Overweight children tend to grow up to be overweight adults and are at much greater risk for obesity-related medical conditions, like diabetes, fatty liver disease, high cholesterol, heart disease, and high blood pressure.

Why Is Obesity a Problem?

THE PHYSICAL EFFECTS

Today children and adolescents spend a great deal more time inside on the computer or in front of the television than in years past. In fact, 43 percent of adolescents watch more than two hours of television each day. Children become less active as they move through adolescence, and inactivity is more common in females (14 percent inactive) than males (seven percent inactive). Black females are reported inactive 22 percent of the time, compared to 12 percent in white females.

THE EMOTIONAL EFFECTS

Being overweight or obese puts a stigma on a child that is difficult to escape. Social discrimination and teasing by peers and family members are immediate results. Studies show that "quality of life" surveys made by obese children were nearly identical to those of children suffering with cancer and undergoing chemotherapy. An impaired quality of life and constant ridicule puts the child at risk for long-term issues with self-esteem and self-worth.

Helping to Prevent Obesity

Losing weight and maintaining a goal weight is difficult for children and adolescents, so the goal must be to prevent the child from becoming overweight. If the child appears to be eating and exercising normally, but still continues to gain weight, it is important to schedule a doctor's visit to determine the cause. There may be a treatable medical condition, like polycystic ovary disease or diabetes, to blame. Of utmost importance is letting the child know they are loved and appreciated just as they are. Here are some ways to keep your child's weight down:

■ Encourage participation in school-based physical education or after-school athletic programs. If your child notices your interest in a particular sport, it may motivate her to give it a try.

■ Make concrete attempts to get the entire family outside for exercise at least once a week. Even a half-hour walk together can get muscles moving and help burn calories.

■ Encourage children to eat only when they are hungry and have healthy, low-calorie snacks available.

■ Be a proper role model. It may be tempting to hit the recliner after work, but think how much better it would be to spend an hour outside walking with your child or throwing a baseball.

■ Reduce the amount of time your child spends in front of the television, computer, or video games.

■ Work with your child's school system to discourage high-calorie, high-sugar drinks and snacks in the vending machines. Send fruit as a snack for late afternoons and opt for healthy, low-fat menus at home.

■ Limit the fast-food fallback by planning meals ahead of time.

DEVELOPING GOOD EATING HABITS

Here are a few additional tips on good eating habits that will help prevent obesity:

■ **Eat only when hungry.** Overeating is one of the most common and dangerous dietary habits. Eating small meals, several times a day, instead of one or two large meals might be a better fit for your child.

■ **Eat slowly.** Chewing food properly allows the digestive process in the mouth to begin. This saves a lot of wear and tear on the stomach and digestive tract, helping us easily break down the food and make the best use of the nutrients contained in it.

■ **Don't undereat.** All forms of undereating like skipping meals or eating only limited foods will lead to inadequate vitamin and mineral levels for proper growth.

■ **Don't eat late.** Eating late can add pounds. Plan early dinners and limit snacks after 9 p.m.

■ **Eat with the stomach, not the emotions.** Our emotions strongly influence our eating behavior. Some children eat when they are upset or depressed; others cannot eat at all in this condition. Watch carefully to observe what emotional factors might influence your child.

■ **Sit down to eat.** Family dinners may be difficult to schedule, but they give everyone the chance to get the most out of the food and the company.

The Nutritional Needs of Children

Research has shown that there is a crucial relationship between nutrition and health and learning ability. There is compelling evidence that diet-related diseases don't necessarily wait until our later years to get their start. Many children typically consume more calories than they expend, which can lead to obesity. Many children eat more fat, saturated fat, cholesterol, and sodium than is recommended and eat too few grains, vegetables, and fruits.

Children need a wide variety of vitamin-containing foods for proper growth and development. Many vitamins are best absorbed and utilized by the body when taken near a mealtime. Listed here are 11 essential vitamins, their benefits to the body, and what foods they are normally found in.

■ **Vitamin: Vitamin A/Beta Carotene**

BENEFITS: Supports the immune system, acts as an antioxidant, and promotes proper cell development. Important for the formation of strong bones and teeth.

FOUND IN: Fish liver oils, animal livers, and green and yellow fruits and vegetables.

■ **Vitamin: Vitamin B-1/Thiamine**

BENEFITS: Supports energy and circulation, helps maintain a healthy heart, and supports a healthy nervous system.

FOUND IN: Dried beans, brown rice, egg yolks, fish, organ meats, soybeans, and whole grains.

■ **Vitamin: Vitamin B-2/Riboflavin**

BENEFITS: Helps promote the health of skin, nails, hair, and vision. Excellent for athletes to provide antioxidant protection. Aids with the metabolism of carbohydrates, fats, and proteins.

FOUND IN: Beans, cheese, eggs, fish, meat, milk, poultry, spinach, and yogurt.

■ **Vitamin: Vitamin C**

BENEFITS: Helps support a healthy immune system, protects against the harmful effects of pollution, promotes healthy bones, and provides antioxidant effects.

FOUND IN: Green vegetables, berries, citrus fruits, mustard, green and sweet peppers, persimmons, tomatoes, turnip greens, and watercress.

■ **Vitamin: Vitamin B-3/Niacin**

BENEFITS: An essential vitamin to help support the nervous system, circulation and a healthy heart.

FOUND IN: Beef, broccoli, carrots, cheese, corn flour, eggs, tomatoes, and whole wheat.

■ **Vitamin: Vitamin E**

BENEFITS: Helps protect the body against free radicals and provides antioxidant effects. Supports a healthy heart and helps promote hormonal balance.

FOUND IN: Cold-pressed vegetables like olive oil and sunflower oil, nuts, seeds, legumes, and eggs.

■ **Vitamin: Vitamin D**

BENEFITS: Supports the immune system, helps promote healthy bones, and helps the body absorb calcium.

FOUND IN: Fish liver oils, dairy products, alfalfa, butter, cod liver oil, egg yolk, salmon, and sweet potatoes.

■ **Vitamin: Vitamin B-12**

BENEFITS: Supports energy functions and promotes a healthy nervous system. Aids with digestion and food absorption.

FOUND IN: Various cheeses, clams, eggs, kidney, liver, seafood, and tofu.

■ **Vitamin: Biotin**

BENEFITS: Helps maintain the health of the hair, skin, and scalp. Aids with cell growth and fatty acid production in the metabolism of carbohydrates, fats, and protein.

FOUND IN: Cooked egg yolk, saltwater fish, meat, milk, poultry, soybeans, whole grains, and yeast.

■ **Vitamin: Folic acid**

BENEFITS: Helps maintain female reproductive health, particularly during childbearing years.

FOUND IN: Barley, beans, beef, bran, brown rice, milk, liver, oranges, tuna, salmon, root vegetables, and yeast.

■ **Vitamin: Vitamin B-6/Pyridoxine**

BENEFITS: Helps support the immune system and the skin and eyes. Activates many enzymes and aids with B-12 absorption.

FOUND IN: Brewer's yeast, carrots, chicken, eggs, fish, sunflower seeds, walnuts, and wheat germ.

■ **Vitamin: Vitamin B-5**

BENEFITS: Provides support for the adrenal glands, digestive tract, and immune system. Also helps promote relaxation and provides mood support.

FOUND IN: Beans, beef, eggs, saltwater fish, mother's milk, pork, fresh vegetables, and whole wheat.

VITAMIN SUPPLEMENTS

Vitaball

A vitamin in a gumball? How neat is that! These taste like real gumballs, but contain 100 percent of the (recommended daily allowance) RDA of vitamins. For adults and children over the age of five, it is necessary to chew one gumball daily. The gumball may be too large for children under the age of five. Parents should supervise children's use. Your child should chew the gumball for five to ten minutes to ensure the release of vitamins.

L'il Critters Gummy Vites Kids

For those little guys who like gummy bears, these are great. As a dietary supplement, parents may give each child up to two L'il Critters

A Drug Lady Reminder

Keep children's vitamins far from little hands. Many of these look and taste like candy, so it is especially important to treat these like any other medicine. An overdosage of some vitamins can be fatal to a child's system.

Gummy Vites per day. These don't contain the full spectrum of vitamins found in most children's multivitamins, but are better than no supplementation at all.

Centrum Kids Complete

This one contains more vitamins and minerals than any other leading complete children's chewable vitamin, (such as Flintstones and Bugs Bunny). Centrum Kids Complete has the Rugrats characters that kids love, plus three great-tasting flavors—cherry, orange, and fruit punch.

Poisons and Home Dangers

There is nothing more important than the safety of your child. Spending time educating them and yourself about the dangers of poisons and other home hazards can be a positive experience for everyone. There are probably some things in your home that you had no idea were dangerous to your children; others are more obvious. Keeping your home safe requires thought and preparation as your infant grows into an inquisitive toddler, and continues through the school and teen years. When your children make their own homes, they'll take the good habits of avoiding home dangers with them to protect those adorable grandchildren.

Poison Proofing the Home

The neighbor child found some medicine in a drawer and ate it. The family spent several scary hours in the emergency room. She's fine now, but I want to be sure that the same thing doesn't happen in our home.

Every year poison control centers receive over one million calls for accidental poisonings of children under the age of five. The majority of these calls are due to medicines and household chemicals. Poisoning isn't something any of us like to think about, but being prepared is the best defense. Remember that packaging that is child-resistant isn't necessarily childproof. Medicines, vitamins, chemicals, and toxic household products should be kept locked up.

Your child will be in the care of others, as well as yourself. It is a good idea to be sure everyone is aware of what to do when there is an emergency. Posting a list of emergency numbers for the grandparents, for the baby-sitter, and for quick access by each telephone is a good start.

An invaluable lesson for every child is getting to know the ugly "Mr. Yuk." Take a safety tour of the house with your young child and put a "Mr. Yuk" sticker on all household chemicals and items that could harm a child if ingested.

Another good idea is putting a sticker by the phones with the number for Poison Control. Most pharmacies and pediatrician offices will be glad to give out the stickers. Poison Control has a national number you can call from anywhere, which will connect you to the closest office. The number is 1-800-222-1222. This is one number worth committing to memory.

If you even suspect that your little one has gotten into something that could be harmful, make the call! Also grab the substance that was swallowed and bring it with you if you go to the hospital. The Poison Control center will ask you a few standard questions to give guidance on what to do next, including the following:

■ What is your child's age and weight?

■ How was the poison taken? Was it swallowed, breathed in, or splashed on the skin or in the eyes?

■ What is the name of the poison?

■ Do you know how much was swallowed?

■ How long ago was it swallowed?

■ Has your child vomited?

■ What symptoms is your child experiencing?

The people at Poison Control are wonderful. They can walk you through exactly what to do and when to seek immediate medical attention. Poison Control can also identify most medicine tablets if your child has taken something and you're unsure of exactly what it is.

An alert parent generally knows when their child is acting strangely. If an opened or spilled bottle of pills is seen, look for these symptoms of poisoning in your child:

■ Acting sleepy or groggy when it's not a normal bedtime.

■ Having difficulty following you with their eyes.

■ Feeling nauseous or vomiting without other signs of illness.

■ Eyes are going around in circles and aren't focusing.

■ Difficulty breathing.

■ Burns or stains around the mouth or excessive drooling.

■ Strange-smelling breath.

The scariest and most dangerous products around the house are drain cleaners, insecticides, and furniture polish. Medicines can also be dangerous. Lock them away and under child-resistant caps at all times.

Hidden Poisons in the Home

We like to think of our homes as a safe place to be. Unfortunately, numerous products in a typical home are possible poison dangers for children. Many things we, as adults, use safely every day can be life-threatening if swallowed by a small child.

One of the biggest hidden poison hazards is the accidental overdose of iron-containing vitamins. Iron-containing supplements are the leading cause of poisoning deaths for children under six in the United States. The scary part is some of the children who died from overdose consumed as few as five pills. Keep vitamins away from a young child in a locked cabinet and don't refer to them as candy for older children; stress the importance of only taking one tablet a day in the presence of a parent. Always close the vitamin container immediately after use and put it away where the child can't reach it. Out of sight is best.

Other seemingly innocent things in the home can also cause poisoning if eaten. Art supplies, lamp oil, candles, houseplants, antifreeze, cigarette butts, paint thinner, and alcohol are all potential poisons to a child.

Lead poisoning from lead-based paint or improperly fired ceramic ware is still a concern in many areas. Children suffer from lead poisoning the most, absorbing up to 50 percent of the lead they ingest. Apartments and homes built before 1978 may have been painted with lead-based paints. Chips and dust from this paint can lead to toxic levels in a child's system. Ceramics bought abroad should not be used for food storage in any way. Cups and pitchers may be especially dangerous for releasing small amounts of lead if hot, acidic foods are put inside. Because the symptoms of this type of lead poisoning aren't usually visible until the damage has been done, a doctor can perform a blood test if you have reason to believe the child was exposed to lead.

A Drug Lady Reminder

Make a "Safe House" list of products that could be harmful to your child. Spend a Saturday morning walking through the home and identifying hidden as well as obvious poison opportunities. You'll be surprised at what you find. Then take steps to put these things out of reach of young hands.

Ipecac Syrup

All of the baby books say to have a bottle of ipecac syrup on hand. However, I've read lately that it isn't good to use. What is ipecac syrup and what does it do?

For many years, this was one of those essentials that every home with a youngster who just might come into contact and swallow something poisonous should have in an easily accessible place. Today, however, the Food and Drug Administration, American Academy of Pediatrics, and American Association of Poison Control Centers are changing their minds. Because of high levels of abuse of this over-the-counter product by those with the eating disorder bulimia as well as studies that it may be effective in only a very small portion of childhood poisonings, ipecac syrup may be on its way out of the baby books forever.

Ipecac syrup is a rather unpleasant-tasting liquid made from plant extracts that stimulates the brain to tell the stomach it's time to throw up. Vomiting usually occurs in 20 minutes or less.

Poison specialists have generally recommended keeping a bottle of ipecac syrup on hand, but not to induce vomiting until the doctor or Poison Control gives the okay. There are some poisons that should not be brought back up because they can severely burn the throat or become aspirated into the lungs. Also, if it's been over an hour after the child swallowed the substance, making him throw up probably won't be helpful.

If it's an acid or caustic substance that was swallowed, like drain cleaner or bleach, the child should *not* be encouraged to throw up. Instead, milk or water will help flush the esophagus. The child should be kept in a sitting or standing position to prevent the poison from coming back up. Petroleum products such as gasoline, lamp oil, or charcoal lighter fluid also should not be vomited back up. Milk or bread already around the house can be used to absorb the substances that have been swallowed and can't be brought back up.

Ipecac syrup is certainly losing favor at Poison Control centers across the country. In 2002, there were 16,000 cases of ipecac treatment for poison ingestion, down from 150,000 in 1986. For certain cases, such as if a child lives hours away from hospital care, ipecac syrup may be a lifesaver. Always call Poison Control to be sure. If the Poison Control center or doctor says it's okay to induce vomiting, give one tablespoonful of ipecac syrup for kids one to six, and two tablespoonfuls for those over six. The dose for infants six to 12 months is two teaspoonfuls. Keep the child walking and give at least six ounces of water to wash down the ipecac. Vomiting should start in 20 minutes, but if it hasn't, go ahead and administer another tablespoonful of ipecac.

Check the expiration date on your ipecac syrup bottle. It isn't effective after it's expired. It is also strongly recommended that you take the child to the hospital even after giving ipecac. The reasoning is that ipecac removes only 30 to 50 percent of the ingested substance, leaving a great deal of poison still in a small body.

For a safer alternative to ipecac, activated charcoal should be another staple in your poison-protecting arsenal. Activated charcoal works by absorbing the poison within the body, making it less harmful. Again, this agent isn't appropriate for all poisons, so only use with the approval of the doctor or the Poison Control center.

Childproofing the Home

I'm a soon-to-be Dad who wants to make sure that everything is perfect before the baby gets here. Any tips on what we should do to have a completely safe childproof home?

First, congratulations new Dad-to-be! A new baby will change your life in ways you never dreamed possible. Get used to not being able to open the cabinet doors or toilet seats for a while! Forget being able to plug in the laptop at a whim and don't even think about leaving those beautiful crystal vases within arms' length for a few more years. There is much to do to get ready for a new baby. An accident can happen in an instant, so instead of worrying about the "what ifs," take the steps now to ensure that your home is as safe as possible.

FOR THE PARENTS
Often, in an effort to make everything perfect for the baby, things are forgotten that are just as important for the parents. Here are a few tips to make the home safer for Moms and Dads:

■ Install night-lights from your bedroom to the baby's room. This will give your feet a clear path to follow in the middle of the night when your brain has not quite engaged.

■ Position the furniture in your new baby's room to be easily accessible in the dark. Practice turning out the light before the baby arrives to see if there are things you may bump into before you find the crib.

FOR THE BABY

Keeping things away from little hands and mouths is important. Remember that everything that the hand can touch will more than likely go into the mouth. Also consider the following tips:

■ Use the crib as a changing table. Often the child feels more secure there and this may prevent a fall.

■ Because your child will be spending a lot of unsupervised time in a crib, please make absolutely sure that the crib meets or exceeds all safety standards.

■ Keep talc powders and lotions far away from little hands, mouths, and noses.

FOR THE TODDLER

Once a toddler is mobile, everything is fair game. It's a good idea to sit down on the floor of each room and take a "toddler's eye view." You'll be surprised at what looks interesting from down there! Also take the following precautions:

■ Tie up cords dangling from curtains and blinds. Cut the loops for extra safety. Children become tangled in the cords and can strangle themselves in just a few minutes.

■ Use covers in all electric outlets. These are available in most baby or hardware stores. It's really not difficult to take these out to plug in the vacuum. Just remember to put them back in!

■ Take a close look at the height of those sharp corners on furniture and remember that falling is a way of life as toddlers learn to walk and run. Replace potentially dangerous furniture, or get corner covers to protect delicate little heads.

A Drug Lady Reminder

One of the most important rules: don't leave the little one unsupervised—even for "just a few minutes." Those little guys and girls are very quick and they move like little magnets toward anything that isn't good for them or is downright dangerous. All of the childproofing in the world won't be effective if they grab something that can harm them. Keep a safe home and a happy little one!

■ Electrical cords look like a wonderful thing to chew on when a toddler is just growing teeth. Keep these up out of reach as much as possible and keep an eye on little crawlers.

■ Don't underestimate the curiosity of a toddler. Just because it's high up doesn't mean they won't climb to get to it. Be sure that bookcases and entertainment centers are secured to the wall.

12

Sunburn, Sunscreens, and Sun-Sensitive Medications

Sun Safety

During childhood, a single blistering sunburn can double the risk of cancer later on in life. Moreover, because one person dies from skin cancer every hour, a child's sunburn isn't something to take lightly. Early damage from sun exposure is a preventable problem. On the average, children get three times more sun exposure than adults, and 80 percent of a person's lifetime sun exposure occurs before the age of 18. Regular use of an SPF 15 or higher sunscreen during the first 18 years of life can decrease your child's chance of developing some forms of skin cancer by 78 percent!

Following are steps from the Sun Safety Alliance to provide the highest level of sun safety for your family:

■ Wear protective clothing and hats. Long-sleeved shirts and long pants protect tender skin.

■ Apply broad-spectrum SPF 15 to SPF 30 sunscreen to children six months and older.

■ Limit outdoor activities during peak sun time, which is 10 a.m. to 2 p.m.

■ Protect your child's eyes by having them wear 100 percent UV blocker sunglasses.

■ Beware of surfaces, like snow, sand, water, and concrete, which can reflect damaging rays.

■ Do not leave infants in direct sunlight. Not only does their tender skin burn more easily, but they are more at risk for heat exposure injuries because their bodies handle heat less efficiently—they sweat less, they generate more heat during movement, and their cardiovascular systems aren't as efficient. Flushed faces, excessive sweating, irritability, restlessness, shaking, and cramps are signs of heat illness. The faster you cool off your child with air conditioning, ice packs, or fans, the better. (See also Heat Stroke, pg. 246.)

Sunburn

The sun naturally produces both UVA and UVB rays. UVA rays cause skin aging and the UVB rays cause burns. Typically, the redness and pain of sunburn will appear in one to 20 hours after the exposure. Fever, nausea, prickly sensations, and chills often come with a more serious sunburn. Small blisters and a lizard-like peeling of the skin as the burn begins to heal are also common. The very best treatment of sunburn is preventing it from happening in the first place.

If a sunburn does occur, cool baths and cool compresses are wonderfully soothing for sun-reddened skin. Orange juice high in vitamin C helps to give the body extra immune support while healing. The aloe plant, and the even handier jar of aloe, is as good for sunburn as for other burns (see Burns, pg. 169). Aloe gel, the jelly-like material found within the leaves of the plant, is thought to work in two ways: First, the compounds in the gel limit the effects of bradykinin, a pain-producing agent in our bodies. Second, it stimulates skin cell growth, immune response, and regeneration of some type of nerve cells.

Help for minor sunburn pain is probably already in your medicine chest. Anti-inflammatory pain relievers, like children's ibuprofen, work well to ease the pain. Children's Tylenol (acetaminophen), while not an anti-inflammatory, is effective for simple pain relief. Cooling sprays, like Solarcaine, contain the numbing agent benzocaine, and are wonderful for those burns when your child can't bear for you to touch the sunburn to apply a cream or lotion.

Sunscreens

Picking a good sunscreen is a little like picking apples; the perfect one depends on what type you are looking for. What looks good for Mom and Dad may not be the best for the little guys. When picking a sunscreen, you should keep in mind factors like the amount of time in the water, the amount of activity, and the time of day your children go out in the sun. A sunscreen arsenal may consist of several different types, and that's fine. It's better to be prepared than to risk a painful and skin-damaging burn. Apply sunscreen on dry skin 15 to 30 minutes before going out into the sun.

Water-resistant and sweat-proof are terms that are commonly attached to sunscreens. Water-resistant simply means that it won't wash off as readily when the kids are in the water. The directions still recommend reapplying every 15 minutes while they're in the water. Remember, just because it says water-resistant doesn't mean a child can swim indefinitely without putting more on. Water-resistant technically should stay effective for up to 80 minutes in the water, but applying more often won't hurt. Every hour while swimming or perspiring heavily is recommended.

Sweat-proof sunscreens typically are a little more binding to the skin. Older children over the age of 12 who play sports in the sun may use these because even after a grueling game of beach volleyball, the sunscreen is for the most part still there. Sweat-proof sunscreens have a greater tendency to clog the pores and actually prevent a child from sweating. Be aware of this and be sure to keep your child's body as cool as possible when using a sweat-proof sunscreen. These aren't recommended for young children. Even this type of sunscreen requires regular reapplication for maximum protection.

To avoid skin irritation, try any sunscreen on a small area of your child's skin first, especially if she has had skin allergies in the past. Because the UVA rays are known to be damaging to the skin (for wrinkles and aging), many products now contain UVA and UVB blockers. These are called broad-spectrum sunscreens.

For the little ones, look for waterproof brands like Waterbabies by Coppertone. This contains skin protectants that have been shown to be safe for delicate skin. These products also come in helpful colors to ensure comple coverage even at the top of the ear and tip of the nose.

Sunscreens come in many forms: creams, gels, sprays, lotions, dab-on sticks, or roll-ons. Be aware of products with high alcohol content, like gels, as these can be drying on the skin and may sting if accidentally placed in the eye.

SPF

SPF stands for "sun protection factor" and it determines a sunscreen's ability to protect the skin against damage from the sun's UVA and UVB rays. It's important to pick the right SPF for everyone in the family. The SPF is a very individual type of ranking. If your child has very fair skin or skin that hasn't seen the sun in a while and normally starts to burn in about 15 minutes, an SPF of 2 would allow her to stay in the sun for twice as long or 30 minutes. If your child has a darker skin tone and doesn't start to turn red until she's been out for forty-five minutes, then the same SPF of 2 would give her an hour-and-a-half in the sun.

An SPF of 2 means that 50 percent of the sun's rays are deflected. An SPF of 15 means that 93 percent are deflected, and an SPF of 30 gives 97 percent deflection. Brands range from SPF of 2 to 60. However, the Food and Drug Administration places a labeling limit of 30+ for any SPF above 30. The American Academy of Dermatology and the National Institutes of Health recommend that everyone start out with an SPF of 15 or higher. The Sun Safety Alliance recommends that children use an SPF of 30.

Sun-Sensitive Medications

Medications and the sun sometimes don't mix. Some medications cause a photosensitivity reaction, meaning that when an individual taking the drug is exposed to sunlight, the skin reacts with a rash, intense burning, redness, and swelling. If your child's degree of sunburn seems out of proportion with the amount of sun exposure, it may be a result of photosensitivity.

There are two types of photosensitivies: phototoxic reactions and photoallergic reactions. Phototoxic reactions may result in a shiny lobster-like redness, or for burns that are more serious, a fever or blisters. Cold compresses and Tylenol (acetaminophen) can be used to treat a milder phototoxic reaction. Photoallergy is a second type of photosensitivity that occurs when the same drugs arouse an immune system reaction. The result is an itchy, raised rash or raised welts. Some sunscreens with PABA trigger a photoallergic reaction.

Following are examples of children's medications that could cause a photosensitizing reaction. There are others, so it is always important to check with the child's doctor or pharmacist about the potential for a reaction when a new medicine is prescribed.

- **Antibiotics/antivirals:**
- Zithromax (azithromycin)

- Zovirax (acyclovir)

- Doxycycline

- Clindamycin

- Tetracycline

- Griseofulvin

- Bactrim, Septra (sulfamethoxazole/trimethoprim)

- Pediazole (sulfisoxazole-erythromycin)

- **Acne:**
- Benzoyl peroxide

- Retin-A (tretinoin)

- **Anti-convulsants:**
- Depakote (divalproex)

- Depakene (valproic acid)

- **Antihistamines:**
- Zyrtec (cetirizine)

A Drug Lady Reminder

Because so many medications can cause sun-induced skin reactions for your child, always ask the pharmacist or doctor about any new medicines before heading off for a vacation at the beach. Often taking a few precautions ahead of time can save days of discomfort later.

- Periactin (cyproheptadine)

- Benadryl (diphenhydramine)

- **Asthma:**
- Azmacort (triamcinolone)

- **Eye Drops:**
- Polytrim (trimethoprim-polymyxin)

PART TWO

Fingertip Advisors

Fast Guidance for Childhood Ailments

ACNE

Acne, or acne vulgaris, as the scientific term implies, is an unpleasant condition. It affects nearly 85 percent of people by the time they are twenty-five years old. The amount of people affected is no consolation, however, when your son or daughter has school pictures or the prom scheduled during a massive outbreak.

Acne is caused by an overproduction of a naturally found skin oil called sebum. The manufacture of too much sebum has been related to an increase of hormones during puberty, certain medications, and even stress. The only acne/fast food connection found so far is from those who work around fryers and are subjected to oil-laden air.

Acne, pimples, or zits are all terms for when sebum causes an oil blockage of skin pores, resulting in inflammation. Bacteria get involved when oil and dead skin become trapped in the pores. Raised red pimples along with whiteheads (total blockage of the pore) and blackheads (partial pore blockage), appear primarily on the forehead, nose, and chin. The neck, shoulders, back, and chest may also be affected.

The key to controlling and eliminating acne in your child is to control and eliminate the things that make it worse. Decreasing sebum production, killing bacteria lying in wait for plugged pores, and removing sloughed off skin cells before they can block pores are all ways of fighting this condition. The severity of the acne outbreak is another major factor in what type of treatment is used.

NATURAL CHOICES
For mild cases of acne, there are several things to try at home.

■ Have your child wash his face in the morning and before bed-time with a gentle soap, which can help remove excess oils, as well as bacteria and dead skin cells.

■ Have your child try a new hairstyle, which may keep the pim-ples away. Hair falling on the forehead and sides of the face has oils that can block pores and make acne worse.

OVER-THE-COUNTER PRODUCTS

One of the most common ingredients in over-the-counter acne prod-ucts is benzoyl peroxide, which can be found in strengths from 2.5 percent up to ten percent. This medicine fights acne in two ways: it kills the bacteria invading those clogged pores and it irritates the skin to such a point that the pores are not able to fully close and become blocked again.

Side effects of benzoyl peroxide include temporary stinging, peel-ing, burning, drying, and redness of the skin. It's best to start with a lower strength and work up to minimize these effects. Because ben-zoyl peroxide depends on a complete turnover of skin, it may take four to six weeks before your child notices the full effects. Zapzyt and Clean and Clear Persa-Gel are both ten percent benzoyl peroxide gels that make the telltale white spots of acne treatment obsolete.

DOCTOR VISITS

For more severe cases of acne or those just not responding to over-the-counter treatment, a doctor's visit is in order. The dermatologist might recommend a combination medicine like BenzaClin topical gel, which contains benzoyl peroxide and the antibiotic clindamycin.

As with over-the-counter products, prescription medications have three goals: to decrease the body's production of sebum, to kill bac-teria, and to keep pores from getting plugged with oils.

Prescription medicines that reduce the amount of sebum made by a person's body are called isotretinoids (Accutane). Accutane is reserved for patients with severe cystic acne that does not respond to other treatments. However, dermatologists must perform a number of blood tests before administering Accutane, and women should *not* get pregnant while taking it due to a high potential for birth defects.

Antibacterial products (antibiotics) can be either applied directly to the face (erythromycin, clindamycin) or taken internally by mouth (minocycline, doxycycline).

Retinoids, like Retin-A (tretinoin), unplug pores by pushing oils and dead skin out from the inside. Retinoids are derivatives of vitamin A. Other retinoids available by prescription for topical skin use are Differin, Azelex, and Tazorac.

ALLERGIC CONJUNCTIVITIS

A diagnosis of conjunctivitis can be confusing. There are actually several different types: allergic, bacterial, and viral. In the allergic variety, caused by pet dander, mold spores, and pollen in the air, the membrane covering the eyeball and the inner eyelid (called the conjunctiva) becomes inflamed. Allergic conjunctivitis typically presents itself as red, itchy, swollen whites of the eyes. Tears may flow and noses may run, but there is no specific infection present, just an allergy. Allergic conjunctivitis usually occurs around the same time as other seasonal allergies. Because this condition isn't contagious, treatment involves decreasing the annoying symptoms as much as possible.

However, there other causes of conjunctivitis to be aware of, including those caused by a bacterial or viral infection. Bacterial conjunctivitis, also called Pink Eye (see Pink Eye, pg. 274), is diagnosed when a discharge of yellow pus in addition to burning and redness appear in your child's eye. The eye may appear "glued together" upon awakening. Bacterial infections require prescription antibiotic drops or ointments from the doctor for treatment. Viral conjunctivitis causes watery eyes and a thinner mucus discharge. Both bacterial and viral conjunctivitis are highly contagious and can be spread easily from eye to eye or person to person.

NATURAL CHOICES

Because allergic conjunctivitis is typically seasonal, along with other allergies, it is often a self-limiting condition meaning it will end on its own. However, there are a few things you can do to help decrease your child's symptoms:

■ It sounds pretty simple, but have your child regularly wash her hands to help decrease the spread of animal dander or other allergens into the eyes.

■ Caution your teenage girls about the dangers of sharing cosmetics with others, particularly those cosmetics that can find their way into the eyes.

■ Bathe your child's eyes with gentle eyewashes, as these can be effective in removing the foreign allergens that are causing the itching and redness.

■ Gently wipe your child's eyes with clean washcloths. Change the washcloths after each use and wash them well.

■ Keep your child away from the allergens that cause allergic conjunctivitis, like smoke, cat hair, or high pollen counts.

OVER-THE-COUNTER PRODUCTS

For children, common products for allergic conjunctivitis are eye-washes and antihistamines. The Lavoptik Eye Wash comes with a small eye cup to make flushing their eyes easier when the pollen counts are high. Artificial tears also provide an excellent on-demand clearing of itchy eyes.

Antiallergy medicines (antihistamines) are another good therapy for allergic conjunctivitis. These can be taken by mouth (like diphenhydramine or Claritin) and help decrease allergy symptoms. Decongestants (like Afrin Children's Eye Drops) may be put directly into the eye to constrict leaky vessels and decrease runny eyes and noses.

DOCTOR VISITS

When little hands are constantly rubbing fiercely itching eyes, it is possible to tear the delicate eye membranes and allow an infection to develop. With children, this can happen very quickly. For more serious cases of allergic conjunctivitis, the doctor may prescribe an antibiotic/steroid combination, like Cortisporin Ophthalmic (polymyxin B, neomycin, and hydrocortisone) to both fight infection and reduce redness and inflammation.

Putting eyedrops into your child's eyes can be a difficult and sometimes frustrating experience. Wasting the drops not only could prolong the condition you're treating, but could also hurt your pocketbook as prescription eyedrops can be *very* expensive.

Here are a few tips:

■ First, wash your hands. It would amaze you how many bacteria are living just on the tip of your finger! You don't want to introduce more bacteria into your child's eyes.

■ Tilt your child's head backward. Try to keep his chin higher than his eyes.

■ Use that freshly washed index finger to pull the lower eyelid away from the eye. See the nice little pouch that forms?

■ Aim the medicine for that pouch. Don't attempt to put the drops directly on the eyeball. That can be very scary and will cause the best of us to blink before that drop hits.

■ Use care not to touch the tip of the dropper to the eyelid.

■ Many eyedrops or ointments can cause blurry vision. This can last for some time after applying them, so inform your child that this may happen and to play quietly until their vision clears.

ALLERGIES

Your child is running around with a perpetually dripping nose and eyes that look as though he's been crying for days. Chances are, he shares one of the most common conditions we know of today: allergies. The difference in an allergy and a cold can be tough to detect. Typically, if your child has allergies, there is a family history of allergies, your child is over two years old, and his symptoms of sneezing, red, itchy, watery eyes, and scratchy throat last for several weeks.

When your child has an allergy, it means that he has developed antibodies against specific allergens, such as pet dander, grass, or pollen. The body sees these allergens as something foreign and dangerous, so the body goes into attack mode to get rid of them. A cycle begins when the eyes water, the nose runs, and your child begins to sneeze.

The first step is to help your child avoid the allergen—that is, whatever triggers the allergy. By reducing your child's exposure to the allergen, you can reduce his symptoms. Because you can't protect your child from all allergens, the second step is to manage the symptoms caused by allergies.

NATURAL CHOICES

To protect your little guys from those annoying allergens, here are a few things to do at home:

■ Use the air conditioner whenever possible.

■ Let someone else comb the dog and cat, then keep your child away for a while after the grooming is done. This ensures the dander will have a chance to settle somewhere other than his nose.

■ Make your home "dust-mite unfriendly." Remove old and musty carpets and vacuum often.

■ Know the pollen counts before he steps outdoors. Encourage inside play on high-count days if possible.

■ Don't use feather pillows as they may initiate sneezes. Look for those products with "hypoallergenic" on the label.

OVER-THE-COUNTER PRODUCTS

Antihistamines, like Benadryl liquid and chewable tablets (diphenhydramine), have been the allergy staple for years. Many doctors still recommend Beradryl as the top over-the-counter product for controlling allergy symptoms. However, newer nonsedating antihistamines like Claritin (loratidine) are now available without a prescription for use in children. The liquid and quick-dissolving Reditabs work well for children over six years old.

Red, itchy eyes can be soothed with a sterile eyewash, like the

Bausch & Lomb brand. Most have special tips or eye cups to help get more of the liquid in the eye than on the clothes.

DOCTOR VISITS

Usually just describing your child's symptoms to the doctor results in a correct diagnosis for allergies, but if the child has trouble breathing or unusual redness around the eyes, it's time for a visit to the pediatrician.

For long-term allergy relief, the physician might recommend a series of allergy shots to allow the child's body to build up immunity against allergens he might come into contact with on a regular basis.

Seasonal allergies may require prescription medicines for the older child. Nasal steroids, like Nasacort AQ (triamcinolone) or Beconase AQ (beclomethasone), help to decrease swelling of nasal membranes and make breathing easier.

ANAPHYLACTIC SHOCK

Anaphylactic shock is a very severe allergic reaction. This condition occurs because of an acute allergic reaction to an allergen the body perceives as foreign. This allergy is much stronger and more intense than the typical allergic reaction. Allergen substances most often causing an anaphylactic reaction are penicillins (and drugs in the penicillin family), medicines containing sulfa, seafood, peanuts, bee stings, and certain vaccines made from horse serums.

Within seconds after exposure to the offending allergen (whether it's penicillin, peanuts, or a bee sting), the body mounts a full assault. The eyes and nose begin to run profusely and swelling occurs on the tongue and throat. Airways close, and it becomes difficult or impossible to breathe. With many children experiencing an anaphylactic reaction, the body may be covered in an itchy rash. Blood vessels begin to release large amounts of fluid into the tissues, dropping blood pressure dramatically. Very low blood pressure means that little oxygen is getting to your child's brain, heart, and other important organs. This fast sequence of events causes a condition called shock.

Unfortunately, this defense system of the body can quickly cause unconsciousness, and if not treated quickly, death. Anaphylactic shock often can be brought on by contact with an allergen that the body has been exposed to previously with no outward effect. This can make a diagnosis tricky.

Symptoms to be aware of are a rapid pulse, difficulty breathing, hives, a swelling of the lips and tongue, damp skin, confusion, or loss of consciousness. If your child shows any of these symptoms, call 911 immediately. Seconds count and a plan in case of such an emergency can make a great deal of difference in the outcome. Spend a few minutes thinking about the logistics of getting your child to medical attention quickly, just in case.

NATURAL CHOICES

The best protection for your family is knowledge and preparation. Know any particular food or drug sensitivities your child has and avoid situations bringing your child into contact with these allergens. Talk to your family doctor, pharmacist, and dentist about any previous drug reactions to avoid a repeat occurrence. Your health care providers can help ensure that nonallergic medications are prescribed and dispensed.

OVER-THE-COUNTER PRODUCTS

The antiallergy product Benadryl (diphenhydramine) should always be in a family's first-aid kit. Benadryl can be taken right after an insect bite or minor allergic reaction to minimize the allergic response. The chewable form is great for storing in your car's glove compartment. While this medication won't halt an anaphylactic reaction, it can buy time until the doctor can be reached. Remember, anaphylactic shock can become life-threatening very quickly. Don't wait to get medical attention.

DOCTOR VISITS

If there is ever a case when a particular allergen provokes a serious reaction, like swelling or extreme itching and redness, an anaphylaxis kit, like EpiPen or EpiPen Jr., should be prescribed by the doctor. Epinephrine is the active ingredient in these lifesaving injection kits. Epinephrine stops cells from releasing histamine, the allergy-causing chemical in the body. It also relaxes the muscles in the throat and airways and tightens the vessels in the nose to allow more free air movement. This medicine works very quickly, often within ten minutes of an injection.

For family picnic or camping trips where medical help may be scarce, always carry—and be certain everyone in the family knows how to use—the EpiPen auto-injector. Spend time with your doctor and pharmacist to be certain you know how to give the potentially lifesaving injection, because once an anaphylactic emergency has begun, it may be difficult to concentrate on reading label directions.

There are two types of EpiPen, the regular (for children over 33 pounds) and the EpiPen Jr. (for children up to 33 pounds). Both are premeasured and preloaded with a small amount of epinephrine. You simply uncap the pen, put the black tip on the thigh, and push firmly. Hold for a count of ten, and then call for additional medical help. According to the package directions, the best spot for an injection is on the outside of the thigh. The quick shot can be done through light clothes and be effective. It is a good idea to practice this series of steps with your children (without administering the actual injection) so everyone is familiar with how to do this in case of emergency.

It is also a good idea to have the child carry a MedicAlert card in their backpack or wear MedicAlert jewelry if there is a history of anaphylactic reactions. It could save their life if they are unable to communicate.

ANEMIA

While there are several different specific forms of anemia—aplastic, megaloblastic, pernicious, sickle cell, and hemolytic—for our purposes, we'll discuss the type most often affecting children, which is called iron deficient anemia. This is the most common type of anemia in the world. Studies have shown that children suffering from acute iron deficient anemia as babies may possibly have lower intelligence levels than those with normal iron counts.

Our bodies use iron as a backbone for hemoglobin, the carrier of oxygen to the brain. Hemoglobin is also the substance that makes our blood red in color. Under the microscope, iron deficient anemia appears as unusually small, pale red blood cells in much lower than normal numbers.

Infants and young children are most at risk as their diets change from iron-fortified formula or breastfed milk to solid food. Their bodies are growing quickly, but their tastes for high-iron foods may not be adequate to supply the body with what it needs. Teenage girls starting menstruation and those worrying about their weight are also commonly at risk for this form of anemia. Symptoms of iron deficient anemia are headaches, pasty skin, pale gums, dizziness, and unusual tiredness. Another low-iron symptom of children is called pica. In this condition, children exhibit unusual cravings for dirt, paint, or ice.

NATURAL CHOICES

The best way to prevent iron deficiency is to ensure your child eats a balanced diet, high in iron-rich foods. Unfortunately, that is often easier in theory than in actual practice. Common foods high in iron content include liver, enriched cereals, red meat, chicken, and fish. Others to try are raisins, dates, dried apricots, nuts, and beans. Tofu and green leafy vegetables are also good choices. Iron is more easily absorbed in the presence of vitamin C, so try adding a glass of orange juice to meals.

OVER-THE-COUNTER PRODUCTS

The recommended daily allowances for iron vary by age and physical condition:

- For infants up to six months: 6mg

- Children six months to ten years: 10mg

- Females 11 to 50: 15mg

- Females over 60: 10mg

- Males 11 to 18: 12mg

- Males 18 and over: 10mg

- Pregnant women: 30mg

A Drug Lady Reminder

WARNING: Iron supplements and vitamins should not be considered candy. In large doses, iron can be very toxic. Poison control reports this as a common cause of fatal overdose among young children. Please keep these out of the reach of children.

A popular liquid supplement for infants and toddlers is Tri-Vi-Sol. This fruit-flavored liquid contains vitamins A, D, and C with 10mg of iron in each dropperful. Many children's chewable vitamins contain iron. Be aware that the side effects of iron may be constipation; dark, hard stools; and stomach upset. These side effects can be lessened by gradually increasing the daily iron dose. Avoid giving dairy products or antacids at the same time as iron supplements, as these can bind with the iron, making it unavailable to the body.

DOCTOR VISITS

If your doctor suspects iron deficient anemia, blood should be drawn for examination. A CBC (complete blood count) will let the doctor know how far along the condition has progressed. Results are typically available within one to two weeks, but you may be advised to start an iron supplement before the diagnosis is confirmed. It can take three to six weeks to turn around iron deficiency anemia, but the supplements are often continued for at least six months to allow the body to replenish its iron stores.

APPENDICITIS

Appendicitis is an often-tricky condition to diagnose at home. It is also potentially deadly. Thankfully, it is rare under the age of two and occurs most commonly in those aged 15 to 30. Noting the symptoms of appendicitis is important and getting prompt treatment could save your child's life.

Appendicitis is an inflammation of the appendix, which is the small area of tissue at the end of the large intestine. The appendix itself is approximately the size of an adult pinkie finger. Once this tissue is inflamed, it fills with bacteria and threatens to burst. If caught in time, the appendix can be removed and the crisis averted. If it bursts, the bacteria are released in the stomach cavity where they can produce a serious infection called peritonitis. Unless treated quickly, peritonitis can be deadly.

Symptoms to be aware of include pain (dull or sharp) along the upper abdominal area around the belly button. It may be sharper toward the right side or the pain may seem to come from the lower abdomen, back, or rectal area. The pain is constant and does not come and go. Your child may have a slight temperature and no appetite. Throwing up may start before the abdominal pain or just after. Swelling of the belly, constipation, or diarrhea are all possible symptoms of appendicitis.

NATURAL CHOICES
If your child shows any combination of the symptoms above, call the doctor. It is best to be overly cautious, rather than risk a ruptured appendix. Avoid giving your child anything to eat or drink until a diagnosis has been made.

OVER-THE-COUNTER PRODUCTS

Over-the-counter products should be avoided if appendicitis is suspected. Laxatives, enemas, and antacids can cause the appendix to rupture. Aspirin should also be avoided, as this could cause blood-clotting problems should surgery be necessary.

DOCTOR VISITS

Symptoms of an appendicitis attack should never be taken lightly. Blood counts are done to determine white cell levels and X rays or a sonogram may be ordered. If appendicitis is suspected, your child will be quickly prepped for surgery. Antibiotics are given as a precaution against bacteria from the inflamed appendix. If it has already ruptured, the abdominal cavity will be cleared of remaining bacteria to reduce chance of infection. The appendix has no known purpose, so once it is removed, your child should suffer no lasting effects other than having a nice scar to show his schoolmates.

ASTHMA

Over 12 million Americans suffer from the lung condition called asthma. Asthma is a constriction or narrowing of the airways leading to the lungs. It is induced by allergic reactions, smoke, cold air, stress, and even exercise. When the airways become irritated, they swell and close, at the same time secreting a sticky mucus substance. What the body is doing is trying to fight off what it sees as a foreign allergen attack by the cold air, exercise, or pollen grains. Higher incidences of allergies and asthma are often seen within families.

Living with asthma can be a difficult situation to deal with, both for the child who suffers from it and for the parent who watches helplessly as their child is unable to take in a breath of air. When the child struggles to breathe, the wheezing and coughing can also be a frightening experience for both child and caregiver. In the past, asthma meant skipping strenuous activities and forgoing sports. Today, however, the asthma diagnosis does not mean the child can't participate. With proper medication and care, an asthma sufferer doesn't have to miss out on any activities.

NATURAL CHOICES
While only prescribed medication can halt an asthma attack, there are things to do at home to ease the stress of asthma:

■ Have your child take a warm, steamy bath, which does wonders to open and soothe inflamed airways. Put a towel over your child's head and have her lean over a big bowl of steamy water for quicker relief.

■ Studies have shown some asthma sufferers to have lower than normal levels of magnesium and B-vitamins. Add supplements to your child's diet to help.

■ Help your child to avoid food allergens, like sulfites or starches, which may trigger an attack. Read product labels carefully.

■ Help your child learn how to avoid and deemphasize stressful situations, which will reduce stress-induced asthma attacks.

■ Identify the triggers that seem to make the condition worse and keep an ongoing diary. Help your child avoid those situations when possible.

OVER-THE-COUNTER PRODUCTS

Because of the seriousness of an asthma condition, most health care providers recommend medical treatment first and the use of other treatments only as a complement to supervised doctor's care. While there are certain products available over-the-counter that are specifically advertised to help with asthma, these may be harmful if not used with appropriate medical care. Very often a first asthma attack will be much milder than progressive ones. Without the proper medicine to help open the airways, your child's life could be in danger.

There are nonmedicinal products that do help the asthma sufferer. A peak flow meter is a device that measures how much the airways are blocked. By exhaling into this handheld meter, you can measure how strongly your child's lungs are able to push air out. Individuals without asthma can empty their lungs of air within three seconds. Asthmatics may take as long as seven seconds to accomplish the same task. By keeping one of these devices at home, you can monitor asthma conditions before they reach a crisis level.

DOCTOR VISITS

Based on your child's symptoms and severity of asthma attacks, the doctor may prescribe one or a series of medications. Prescription treatments for asthma are generally one of three types:

1. Bronchodilators. Bronchodilators open the airways quickly. Bronchodilators, like albuterol (Proventil, Ventolin), ipratropium (Atrovent), or albuterol/ipratropium (DuoNeb), are used for relief during an actual asthma attack. Albuterol and ipratropium are available in a portable inhaler form (MDIs) and in liquid forms for use in the nebulizer (machine that dispenses asthma medication). Albuterol is also available in tablet and syrup form. DuoNeb is for nebulizer use only.

2. Anti-inflammatory Steroids. Anti-inflammatory steroids decrease the swelling in the airways over time. Anti-inflammatory steroids, like Azmacort (triamcinolone) or Flonase (fluticasone), are used to prevent asthma attacks from occurring. These should be used every day and *not* during an actual attack. The medicine in these products acts to prevent the swelling in the airways when your child is exposed to something that could trigger an asthma attack, not when an asthma attack is occurring.

In emergency situations, the doctor may prescribe a stronger steroid like Prelone (prednisolone) to keep the airways open. Generally, this liquid is given in tapered doses—that is, a larger dose on the first day, with the dose gradually decreased or tapered down over the next few days until the asthma is under control. The doctor may prescribe this medicine in combination with one of the bronchodilators, like albuterol, to greatly increase breathing ability.

4. Antiallergy medicines. Antiallergy medicines work by decreasing the allergic reactions that trigger some forms of asthma. Antiallergy drugs, like Claritin (loratidine) or Zyrtec (cetirizine), block the receptors that react to allergic histamines. Because allergies and asthma are so closely connected, preventing the allergy may prevent the asthma attack.

A Drug Lady Reminder

Asthma medicines come in many different forms. One of the most portable ways for older children to carry these medicines with them everywhere is in a metered dose inhaler (or MDI). Here are a few tips for proper MDI use:

1. Shake the MDI several times before starting the puffing procedure. Remove the cap from the mouthpiece to prevent injuries to friends standing close by.
2. Exhale completely, and then hold the mouthpiece about three finger widths from your mouth. Open mouth. Aim. As the breath comes in, press the container and fire.
3. Keep inhaling until the lungs are full. Take a big breath.
4. Hold this for as long as possible. Try counting to five by 1000s— 1001, 1002, 1003, 1004, 1005. Then exhale.
5. If the doctor prescribes more than one puff, wait at least a minute before repeating. Longer than a minute is better, but try to hold off at least for 60 seconds.

ATHLETE'S FOOT

Yes, even full-fledged couch potatoes can contract athlete's foot, which is also referred to as tinea pedis. The fungus responsible for this itchy, scaly, and burning condition of the foot isn't particular.

The fungus looks first for an opportunity to find a home in the moist folds between the toes. The fungus itself goes by the formal names of *Trichophyton* or *Epidermophyton*. It can easily be picked up in the wet areas around pools, showers, and gym locker rooms.

Once it finds a susceptible foot, the fungus thrives in the warm, humid environment provided by socks and tightly fitting shoes. With over 250,000 sweat glands per foot to provide moisture, it's easy to see why athlete's foot is so prevalent. When the fungus finds a home between the toes, it often doesn't stop there. Feeding on the hard outer layer of skin (or keratin), these fungi cause cracks and breaks in the skin, allowing easy access to a secondary bacterial infection on the soles and toes. Intense burning, blistering, itching, foot odor, and peeling of the skin are common symptoms of this annoying condition.

Fortunately, athlete's foot is both preventable and treatable. To prevent the fungus from finding a home between the toes, keep bathroom shower surfaces clean, wear water sandals around crowded pool areas, and most of all keep the feet as dry as possible.

NATURAL CHOICES

Nature produces her own antifungal product called tea tree oil (melaleuca alternifolia). Many pharmacies and health food stores carry this liquid, which has been used for many years as both an antibacterial agent and an antifungal. Look for a 100 percent concentration and be prepared to dab it on the area with a cotton ball or swab twice daily for two to three weeks to ensure complete elimination of the fungus.

A Drug Lady Reminder

WARNING: When using tea tree oil on sensitive little feet, be aware that many brands contain large amounts of alcohol that can sting!

OVER-THE-COUNTER PRODUCTS

When your little one has athlete's foot, it is important to read the over-the-counter package directions carefully as many are age-specific. For children over 12 years old, the fastest over-the-counter treatment to date is Lamisil AT and DesenexMax (terbinafine hydrochloride). The once-a-day for one week dosing is almost twice as fast as other over-the-counter products.

For children over two years, there are several choices for over-the-counter treatment. Tinactin (tolnaftate) both treats and helps prevent recurrence, while Micatin (miconazole) and Lotrimin AF (clotrimazole) cure the fungus in 60 to 70 percent of all cases. Use these twice daily for two weeks.

Now you know what to use, but that's only half the battle. What form do you use? There are solutions, ointments, creams, powders, and sprays all lined up on the shelf. An ointment, liquid, or cream is most effective in getting the medication to the source of the fungus. Powders and sprays are excellent for mild symptoms.

DOCTOR VISITS

For particularly stubborn cases of athlete's foot, it may be necessary for a doctor visit. If redness and itching persist, even after over-the-counter treatments have been tried, the doctor may need to prescribe a more powerful antifungal product, in either oral (by mouth) or topical (directly on the skin) form. The oral products, like Lamisil (terbinafine), Nizoral (ketoconazole), or Sporanox (itraconazole), treat the infection from the inside out, and the side effects may be unsuitable for children. Topical medicines, such as ketoconazole or Lotrisone (clotrimazole/betamethasone dipropionate), may be a better choice for the younger set.

ATHLETIC INJURIES

The top sport injury among schoolchildren is a fracture of the arm or leg. Following closely is knee swelling, muscle strain, ankle sprain, and back/shoulder injury. Every year, over 1,400,000 children under the age of 15 are treated for sports injuries. The decision to allow children to play sports is a good one for both parents and the child. Knowing what steps to take to ensure your child's safety on and off the sports field entails guidance and support for the younger individual.

According to many orthopedic physicians, the majority of sports injuries are preventable as long as the youth is conditioned properly and has regular physical examinations. Whether it's soccer, basketball, in-line skating, snowboarding, or football, even the best-conditioned athlete may suffer an injury. As a caregiver, you will need the knowledge at hand to treat the common injuries, allow the proper time for healing, and ensure the young athlete gets further help when needed.

There are as many different athletic injuries as there are sports to get them in. Injuries to the body from sports almost always involve the bones or the muscles, ligaments, tendons, and tissues surrounding the bones. The structure that transmits the force of the muscle contraction to the bone is called a tendon. When a muscle contracts it pulls on a bone to cause movements. With overuse, the tendon becomes inflamed, tender, and very painful. This condition is called tendonitis.

Ankle sprains are common athletic injuries that occur when ligaments are stretched or torn. A strain occurs when a muscle or tendon becomes slightly overstretched, but doesn't tear.

NATURAL CHOICES

The body is often the best indicator of when it's time to take a break. Children should be encouraged to listen to their bodies. If something hurts or feels funny, the child should stop immediately and seek an adult for help. Learning their physical limits is important while bodies are growing and changing.

One of the basic tenets of sports injury is the R.I.C.E. method. This works best for treating a sprain or strain.

- **R.** Rest. Stop all activity.

- **I.** Ice. Place ice on the injured area (ice packs are great).

- **C.** Compression. Wrap snugly with an elastic bandage (like an ACE bandage).

- **E.** Elevate. Try to keep the injured area higher than your heart. This prevents blood from pooling and decreases swelling.

With children, it is important that proper stretching and conditioning is emphasized. Warmer muscles are less likely to be hurt. For simple sore muscles, a warm soak in the bathtub may bring welcome relief. Sprinkle a cupful of Epsom salt into the water for a soothing effect.

OVER-THE-COUNTER PRODUCTS

For normal muscle strains and sprains, the older child might benefit from an analgesic rub like Icy Hot or Tiger Balm. These cause a burning sensation that increases blood flow to the injured tissue.

Advil (ibuprofen) and Tylenol (acetaminophen) liquids, taken by mouth, are good choices for fast pain relief. Be sure to read the directions carefully as doses vary between different product types.

There will be times when the injury doesn't warrant a doctor's visit, but does require the contents of the first-aid kit. Here are few items you might find necessary:

■ **Bandages.** Bandages are important for covering a wound. These act as a protection against things in the air or from bumping into objects that would hurt. For small cuts or scrapes, a Band-Aid® will cover nicely. If the child has a large wound, it is generally recommended that it not be covered unless it is absolutely necessary. When a bandage is put over a healing injury, it can actually trap bacteria inside and make the healing process take longer. Scars also form much more easily when the area is kept covered and away from the air.

■ **Tape and/or braces.** Tape and/or braces can be used to support a weak area of the body, like an ankle, for instance. Many athletes will put on both a knee brace and tape the knee to both protect and support an old injury.

■ **Splints.** Splints are used to completely immobilize an area of the body. Broken arms are put into a splint until a cast can be put on. Splints are great for small appendages like broken fingers or toes. You would only use a splint on your child when it was important that the injured part of the body not move around. Finger splints are usually made of metal or hard plastic and can be taped for extra support.

DOCTOR VISITS

Obviously, broken bones require immediate attention. However, if your child suffers a sports injury that doesn't look serious at first, but complains of pain for over 12 hours or is unable to use a limb properly, it is advisable to see a doctor as soon as possible. Some fractures can be tricky to detect and may require an X ray for confirmation. Then a cast will be applied to immobilize the injured limb.

Other pains should also be attended to as soon as possible. Your child may be suffering from a severe sprain requiring crutches to prevent further injury.

BAD BREATH

So your child's breath makes your eyes water? It's probably more common than you think. Bad breath, or halitosis, in children can be caused by poor brushing habits, an infection, or those nasty allergies. Bacteria collect on the back of the throat or between the teeth and begin to break down whatever they find there. This results in a foul smell until the problem is cleared up.

Good dental hygiene and proper management of allergy symptoms are generally enough to stop bad breath in its tracks. However, if your child has unusual-smelling breath, like a particularly sweet odor, it's a good idea to let the doctor know so she can rule out any other conditions, like diabetes.

NATURAL CHOICES

Once a more serious cause for bad breath has been ruled out, you can begin concentrating on ways to make brushing the teeth easier for everyone. Here are a few guides for making this a fun time at home:

- Be sure your child's toothbrush fits her mouth. Big brushes can hurt little mouths.

- Let your child pick her favorite brush. If they pick it out, chances are much better that they'll use it.

- Use soft bristles, which are better. Hard bristles can damage tender young gums.

- Make brushing a game. Try putting a kitchen timer by the bathroom sink and see who can keep brushing their teeth the longest. At least three minutes is a good start.

For older children, a tongue cleaner/scraper may be effective. Children should be supervised and shown how to go from the back of the tongue forward, without traumatizing the tongue (and you) in the process.

OVER-THE-COUNTER PRODUCTS

To make brushing more interesting, buy some disclosing tablets. Remember those from elementary school? Have your kids chew on these red tablets and see if there are any red stains left over. Red stains show that plaque is still present and brushing isn't quite doing the job.

Ask your child's dentist about fluoride mouthwashes. These can be used for those over the age of eight who can safely gargle without swallowing the mouthwash.

Children may not like the strong taste of adult toothpaste. Experiment with different kid-friendly toothpastes to find their favorite tastes. Fruit flavors replace the minty taste of adult brands. Barney, Barbie, and Tweetie have gotten into the act with children's toothpastes. Bubble gum, watermelon, and grape are favorite flavors. Instructions for adult-supervised children two years of age and older are; brush teeth thoroughly, preferably after each meal or at least twice a day, or as directed by dentist or physician. For children two to six years; use only a pea-sized amount and supervise the child's brushing and rinsing to minimize swallowing.

DOCTOR VISITS
The American Dental Association recommends that "if marked breath odor persists after proper toothbrushing, the cause should be further investigated" by a physician or dentist. There could be other reasons for your child's foul breath, including sinusitis, postnasal drip, tonsillitis, tooth decay, or objects inserted into the nose.

BEE STINGS

Children enjoy playing outdoors right in the center of many insects' natural habitat. Stings don't only come from bees, but from yellow jackets, hornets, fire ants, and a host of flying and crawling bugs.

For most children, a bee sting or insect bite is a source for mild alarm, with them experiencing an initial sharp pain, followed by mild swelling and itching of the bitten area. If the stinger is still visible (as with a honeybee sting), scrape it away carefully with a knife or a fingernail. Removing the stinger as quickly as possible decreases the swelling and redness.

The bite typically causes quite a bit of pain itself, but with some people, the reaction is much stronger than just discomfort. Over one million Americans are allergic enough to these stings to cause a trip to the emergency room. (See Anaphylactic Shock, pg. 138.)

NATURAL CHOICES

Protect your children outdoors by ensuring that they wear proper clothes to avoid the stings when possible. However, insect bites are often inevitable, so if your child is stung, immediately put ice on the sting area to bring down the swelling. Try to avoid rubbing the area as much as possible, as this will spread the insect's venom.

Try a paste of Adolph's Meat Tenderizer and water directly on the sting. This has been shown to help the pain and itch of a sting. The theory behind using meat tenderizer is that it contains an enzyme called papain that breaks down proteins. Bee venom is a protein, and if this paste of 50/50 water and tenderizer is applied early enough, it can break down the poison before your child's body has a chance to start the allergic reaction process.

OVER-THE-COUNTER PRODUCTS

This is a time where your family's first-aid kit will get good use (see pg. 309). Chewable antihistamines, like Benadryl (diphenhydramine), are a good choice to decrease itching. Calamine lotion or hydrocortisone cream, applied directly to the bite, will also quickly decrease the urge to itch. Tylenol (acetaminophen) can be used to relieve the pain and discomfort of the sting. Both liquid and tablet forms are available.

DOCTOR VISITS

If the insect sting provokes a serious reaction, such as breathing difficulty, swelling, or extreme itching and redness, an immediate trip to the doctor's office is in order. After the bite is treated by antihist-

A Drug Lady Reminder

After Bite KIDS is a great product to apply just after the bite. Touted as a nonstinging itch eraser, this cream also provides the natural antiseptic tea tree oil. It's specifically advertised for children two and over. For those under two, ask your doctor.

amines, an anaphylaxis kit should be prescribed by the doctor. The medicine in these injection kits is called epinephrine. Epinephrine stops cells from releasing histamine, the chemical that causes the problems in an allergic reaction. It also relaxes the muscles in the throat and airways and tightens the vessels in the nose to allow more free air movement. This medicine works very quickly, often within ten minutes of an injection.

If you or your family has a history of allergic reactions, it is very important to always carry a small anaphylactic kit (like EpiPen or AnaKit) for the "just in case" situations. These contain an injection you and all family members can learn to quickly inject until medical help arrives for the allergic individual (see p. 140). It is also a good idea to have the child carry a MedicAlert card in their backpack or wear MedicAlert jewelry if there is a history of anaphylactic reactions. It could save their life if they are unable to communicate.

BEDWETTING

Bedwetting, also called primary nocturnal enuresis, is defined as urination during the hours of sleep in children older than seven or eight years. It is cause for concern if it happens at least twice a week for at least three months and is affecting the child's performance in school or self-esteem.

The cause may be one or several of these factors:

■ A lack of the hormone ADH, the antidiuretic hormone regulating how much urine the body produces.

■ A small bladder capacity, making an eight-hour sleep without urination impossible.

■ A development and growth that may be behind others of the same age.

■ An ability to sleep so soundly and deeply that the child doesn't feel the urge to empty his bladder.

For five to seven million American children over the age of six, bedwetting is a real problem. Social activities are limited, a full night's rest is impossible, and conflict develops with siblings and sometimes with sleepy parents. It is important to understand that the child isn't doing this out of an attempt at misbehaving. He has a medical problem, that when tackled with knowledge and the right tools, is typically cured within 12 to 14 weeks.

NATURAL CHOICES

There are positive steps to be taken at home to ensure the child's self-esteem is preserved and family harmony is kept intact:

- Limit the child's liquids at night, especially caffeine-containing beverages like sodas or tea.

- Establish a bedtime routine that includes a trip to the bathroom.

- Set up a reward system for dry nights.

- Have a set of dry sheets or a sleeping bag near the bed, so the child can take responsibility for changing his own bed.

- For nights when accidents do occur, avoid blaming the child. Remember, this isn't happening because the child is doing it on purpose; it is a normal part of growing up.

OVER-THE-COUNTER PRODUCTS

There are several effective alarm systems for helping children get through the bedwetting crisis. The Wet-Stop alarm is a small, wearable alarm that helps children learn to achieve nighttime dryness by conditioning the child to stop the flow of urine when sleeping. A buzzer sounds at the first drops of urine and awakens the child.

However, an alarm alone won't solve the problem. Parents play an important role in helping their child wake up when the alarm goes off. Because of their child's deep sleep, many parents hear the alarm before their child responds to it. By reminding the child what to do next—go to the bathroom to urinate—the parents help to establish a new response. Over a few weeks to months, the child learns to do this on her own.

DOCTOR VISITS

Medications for bedwetting may be prescribed for several reasons:

■ For children over the age of eight who are having difficulty controlling nighttime wetting or those for whom other treatments have failed.

■ If the child is going away to camp or overnight activities and needs extra help to ensure less chance of embarrassment.

■ In conjunction with other treatments, like the wearable alarm system.

For children who fit into one of these cases, the doctor may prescribe DDAVP (desmopressin). This drug is similar to the natural antidiuretic hormone in the body that the child may be lacking. DDAVP works by decreasing the body's production of urine.

For children with an overactive or small bladder as the cause of the problem, Ditropan (oxybutynin) is often prescribed. Children who are using a combination of bedwetting alarms and medication may be prescribed a medicine called Tofranil (imipramine). Imipramine keeps the child from reaching the deepest stages of sleep where they are unaware of the bladder feeling full.

BLISTERS

A blister is easy to identify. Look for a red, painful area of skin with a bubble of fluid buildup underneath. Blisters aren't all bad. They are part of the body's natural defense system. They are typically caused by friction of something rubbing against the skin, such as a new or ill-fitting shoe, or socks that slip and slide. Blisters form a liquid-filled bubble under the skin for protection against this friction. Unfortunately, blisters really hurt, especially if they happen to pop.

Blisters on the skin can also be caused by burns or allergies. Small blisters on the fingers and cuticles may signal an infection.

NATURAL CHOICES

To prevent blisters, soft, nonrubbing shoes at school are a must. Allowing your child to go barefoot around the house will also help decrease blisters from shoes. For those times when more structured shoes are a must and walking or running is imperative, putting on two pairs of socks with talc powder between them can be effective as blister prevention.

If a friction blister develops, the best healer is time and eliminating friction until the skin underneath has a chance to form and toughen. Due to the risk of infection, popping a blister is not a good idea. Opening the top layer of skin can allow bacteria to reach the delicate skin under the blister and a painful infection could develop. If left alone, the liquid will reabsorb and the blister will heal on its own. If the blister should break open, clean the area gently with soap and water and cover with a bandage.

OVER-THE-COUNTER PRODUCTS

Moleskin is a spongy, flannel material that can be found in the foot-care aisle and applied directly over and around the blistered area. Covering the area with this will protect the area and keep direct friction to a minimum. For hardened skin around a blister, dab on a small amount of Vaseline, which will keep the skin soft and pliable.

If the blister bursts, you should apply a topical skin antibiotic like Neosporin or Polysporin to the area. Antibiotics kill existing bacteria

A Drug Lady Recommendation

One product I like is Blister Relief from Band-Aid. It covers the blister completely and protects it from any more irritation. The adhesive seals it completely, and when it is removed after 48 hours or when the patch becomes loose, the blister is almost completely healed.

and help protect from a bacterial infection developing. Once the over-the-counter antibiotic has been applied, cover the area with a bandage. Topical over-the-counter antibiotics, like bacitracin, neomycin, and polymyxin B, should be used only on fresh wounds, not those that are already infected. Call the doctor just to be sure.

DOCTOR VISITS

If you notice a blister on your child that contains white or yellow liquid or that refuses to go away and looks unusually red and irritated, he may have an infection that should be treated with oral antibiotics, like amoxicillin. Call the doctor to have a look if anything about the blister appears unusual or if the blister takes longer to heal than normal.

BOTULISM

This is a specific form of food poisoning (see Food Poisoning, pg. 233) that is caused by the nasty *Clostridium botulinum* bacterium. This bacterium can be found anywhere, but it especially likes tightly closed home-canned jars of food and vegetables that haven't been properly heated. When the spores of the *Clostridium botulinum* bacteria are consumed, they grow in the intestines and release a toxin that causes botulism. Of the 120 botulism cases reported each year, nearly three-fourths are infants who get it from improperly prepared honey. All forms of botulism can be fatal.

The classic symptoms of botulism are nausea, vomiting, diarrhea, and stomach pain followed in 12 to 48 hours by double vision, blurred vision, drooping eyelids, slurred speech, difficulty swallowing, dry mouth, and muscle weakness.

Infants with botulism appear lethargic, feed poorly, are constipated, and have a weak cry and poor muscle tone. These are all symptoms of the muscle paralysis caused by the bacterial toxin. If untreated, these symptoms may progress to cause paralysis of the arms, legs, trunk, and respiratory muscles. In food-borne botulism, symptoms generally begin 18 to 36 hours after eating a contaminated food, but they can occur as early as six hours or as late as ten days.

NATURAL CHOICES

Avoid giving infants raw honey or home-canned foods. Babies and toddlers should not receive unpeeled or unwashed raw or uncooked foods.

Some common botulism culprits include home-canned foods with low acid content, such as asparagus, green beans, beets, and corn. If home-canned foods are served to the family, be sure they are heated to at least 180° F for ten to 15 minutes. Containers where pickling or canning occurs should be sterilized in boiling water.

To reduce the risk of botulism when pickling food, foods should be washed and cooked adequately. Hands, utensils, containers, and other surfaces that encounter food should be cleaned with soap and warm water.

OVER-THE-COUNTER PRODUCTS

Because of the deadly potential of this toxin, over-the-counter products should not be used for treatment. Prompt medical attention is required.

DOCTOR VISITS

Any family member who develops symptoms of botulism should be seen right away by a health care provider, who can often make a diagnosis by taking a stool sample. Infants with botulism usually require intensive medical care to help them get through the respiratory paralysis. However, if children receive proper medical attention, they usually recover well. State health departments and the Centers for Disease Control have people knowledgeable about botulism available to consult with physicians 24 hours a day. If an antitoxin is needed to treat a patient, it can be quickly delivered to a physician anywhere in the country.

Botulinum toxin (Botox) is used as a treatment for children with cerebral palsy. When injected into a muscle that is spastic or stiff, it can help to decrease the muscle tone for about four to six months.

BRONCHITIS

Bronchitis is the acute inflammation of the bronchial tree, which are the large tubes carrying air to the lungs. This inflammation causes swelling and a sticky secretion of mucus covering the bronchial tubes. Breathing is challenging, and the sound of wheezing as air comes in and out is often heard. Low-grade fever, cough, and runny nose are also common symptoms that gradually worsen over three to four days. This will typically be followed by a frequent, dry, hacking cough, called a nonproductive cough. As the infection worsens, the cough may become wet and phlegmy, which is called a productive cough. A virus causes most cases of bronchitis, so antibiotic therapies won't be effective. However, symptoms should gradually improve over the next five to ten days.

NATURAL CHOICES

Because your child's little airways are inflamed, it's difficult to breathe in air. Help at home by keeping your child away from smoke. Quiet time should be emphasized, as rest will help the body fight the infection.

Wet, or productive, coughs can be aided by having your child drink lots of liquids. This thins the mucus and makes it easier for your child to bring up phlegm.

OVER-THE-COUNTER PRODUCTS

Cool mist humidifiers are wonderful for soothing irritated airways and easing congestion. They use water at room temperature and push it through a rotating disk to form tiny water droplets. These should be cleaned after every use with a bleach or alcohol mixture to kill bacteria, viruses, or fungi that can find a home there.

Steam vaporizers allow medicines, like Vicks VapoSteam, to be added to the machine for extra cough- and congestion-fighting power. Use care with this type of vaporizer due to the potential for burns from the hot steam.

Over-the-counter pain relievers and fever reducers, like Tylenol (acetaminophen) or Motrin (ibuprofen), can make your child more comfortable. For those nights when a cough is limiting their sleep, an over-the-counter cough suppressant, like Robitussin DM (guaifen-esin/dextromethorphan), may be helpful. These should only be used during the dry, hacking, non-productive cough stage. It controls coughs and loosens and relieves chest congestion. For children aged two to six years, the dose is one-half teaspoonful every four hours. For kids aged six to 12, the dose is one teaspoonful every four hours.

DOCTOR VISITS

A virus causes most cases of bronchitis, so antibiotics won't be effective. The "chest cold" will just have to run its course. However, if the cough is impairing your child's sleep, a doctor's visit would be wise. Cough medications may be prescribed that allow your child to sleep through the night.

See the doctor if your child experiences pain on the side of the chest, blood in the mucus from coughing, or if the bronchitis worsens after three to four days instead of getting better.

BURNS

There are many different types of burns, and knowing the best treatment for the particular type will speed relief for your child if such an accident occurs. There are several possible causes for a burn:

- Steam or hot water (moist heat)

- Chemicals

- Electricity

- A flame or hot stove (dry heat)

- Sunburn

Burns can happen quickly and bring with them a great deal of pain and discomfort. Fast relief is imperative. There are many different ways to cool burns, but before you treat them yourself, be certain it is only a minor burn. Easing the pain is important, but if there is tissue damage, a doctor's care is needed to prevent infection and other complications.

When a child's delicate skin is damaged by a burn, the extent of the damage to the underlying tissue determines the degree of the burn:

- First-degree burns, like sunburn, involve only the top layer of skin (epidermis). This type of burn is characterized by redness and pain, but no blisters.

- Second-degree burns go deeper into the tissue and are accompanied by blistering skin. The pain may be severe.

■ Third-degree burns go through all layers of the skin and destroy nerves, too. There is little pain because the nerves are no longer transmitting impulses. The skin may look charred or it may appear bright cherry red.

Fortunately, 85 percent of burns are of the minor or first-degree variety. This doesn't mean they don't hurt, only that there is less risk for infection and scarring. Prompt medical attention is required for any burns that involve the face, the palms, the soles of the feet, or that occur on someone under the age of two.

NATURAL CHOICES

With a burn, it is important to know what *not* to do. Although your mother may have done it, putting butter, grease, or oil on a burn is not a good idea. These oils seal in bacteria and provide a nice home for a bacterial infection. The skin can't breathe, so the burn feels warm for a longer period.

To instantly cool a minor burn, apply a small ice pack to the area. Make these ice packs quickly at home by filling up a baggie with crushed ice cubes and sealing it shut. For sensitive areas, use a soft cloth barrier between the ice pack and the skin. In a pinch, grab a package of frozen vegetables (peas, corn, broccoli) and use this as an ice pack. Keep this on for at least half an hour or until the pain subsides.

Another product to have in every home with children is aloe. Aloe gel, the jelly-like material found within the leaves of the plant, is thought to work in two ways: First, the compounds in the gel limit the effects of bradykinin, a pain-producing agent in our bodies. Second, it stimulates skin cell growth, immune response, and regeneration of some type of nerve cells. In health food stores or pharmacies, look for "pure gel" rather than "aloe extracts" that may be diluted and not as helpful when they are needed. Pure products do tend to break down fairly quickly, however. It may be necessary to replace these periodically to ensure that you have the highest potency possible.

If someone in your household suffers from a burn, make sure they take extra vitamins and minerals. Vitamin A, beta-carotene, and zinc aid in skin healing. Vitamin C also helps to give the body extra immune support while healing.

OVER-THE-COUNTER PRODUCTS

Cooling sprays, like Solarcaine, contain the numbing agent benzocaine. Some also have a mild antiseptic to help decrease the chances of infection. These products are wonderful for sunburns or mild burns when your child can't bear for you to touch the burned area to apply a cream or lotion.

For fast pain relief, try a liberal application of an aloe vera gel with lidocaine. The aloe vera reduces pain and heals the skin with the added bonus of lidocaine to act as a numbing agent.

Pain relievers of the anti-inflammatory variety, like ibuprofen (Advil, Motrin) or naproxen sodium (Aleve), help ease discomfort while the burn heals. Check age-appropriate dosages among the products. Some are not recommended for younger children.

For first-degree burns in a small area, the application of a thin layer of antibiotic ointment with pain reliever is warranted. The entire area should be covered with a nonstick bandage or gauze, and the dressing changed every one to two days.

DOCTOR VISITS

In cases of more serious burns where the skin is obviously charred or scorched, it is important to get the child to the doctor as soon as possible. To prevent shock, keep the child warm and the burn covered with a clean, damp towel or cloth.

At the doctor's office, burns are treated with the cream Silvadene 1% (silver sulfadiazine). Just a small layer of this cream protects the skin against bacteria and some forms of yeast. However, this cream shouldn't be used if your child has a previous sulfa allergy.

If hospitalization is required, the child may be put on intravenous fluids. Here the physician can assess the skin damage and determine what further care the child will need.

CANKER SORES

Canker sores, also called aphthous ulcers, are small, open wounds in the mouth. They are distinguished from other mouth conditions by the gray membrane covering the ulcer. The edges of the canker ulcer may be bright red and can be very painful. Chewing can be difficult, and consuming acidic foods, like orange juice, can cause agony.

Most children develop these ulcers after biting the inner cheek or lips. Also, rough use of the toothbrush around delicate mouth membranes has been linked to canker sore development. The medical cause is unknown. It may be related to a virus, stress, anxiety, or lack of vitamins. Some studies have even shown that the active ingredient in some toothpastes, a product called sodium lauryl sulfate, may worsen or even cause canker sores to form. Most canker sores heal within two weeks, but for a child in pain, those two weeks can seem like an eternity.

NATURAL CHOICES
Cool, bland foods, like Jell-O, milk, or ice cream, can be tolerated easier than hard-to-chew choices. Children over the age of 7 may be

shown how to rinse their mouths—and not swallow—with a solution of two tablespoonfuls of table salt in a glass of water. This is soothing on the inflamed tissue.

Often simply adding a multivitamin to your child's diet will decrease or even eliminate the canker sore outbreaks. There has been a distinct correlation between low levels of certain vitamins and minerals and more frequent canker sores.

OVER-THE-COUNTER PRODUCTS

For children over the age of seven, a rinse with a diluted solution of two percent hydrogen peroxide can be helpful. In addition, swishing Milk of Magnesia or Maalox in the mouth coats and protects the sores. Be sure they spit out the remainder of the rinse.

For children over three years, try UlcerEase, a medicine that contains glycerin, which protects the sore, and phenol, which fights bacteria. Have your child use full strength as a mouth rinse, rinsing the affected areas for 15 seconds and then expelling the remainder. Relief will occur with first rinsing. Repeat every two hours, or as needed. Each additional rinsing will bring longer-lasting relief. For best results, continue treatment for two days. For children over three years, apply UlcerEase directly to hard-to-reach ulcers with a cotton swab.

Some over-the-counter remedies, like Anbesol, contain a local anesthetic (benzocaine) to relieve pain instantly. Check the packaging for age-appropriate dosing.

DOCTOR VISITS

For children with canker sores that interfere with eating or speaking, it is time to see the doctor. Kenalog in Orabase (triamcinolone) is a topical steroid cream that contains a numbing agent. This sticky paste covers the ulcer and protects the area while it heals. It has to be applied rather often, but offers instant relief.

The soothing Magic mouthwash, a combination product of diphenhydramine, lidocaine, and Maalox, can be prepared by the pharmacist with a doctor's prescription.

CAT SCRATCH DISEASE

Cat scratch disease or cat scratch fever occurs in children bitten or scratched by a kitten or young cat that (while not ill itself) is carrying the *Bartonella henselae* bacteria. This bacteria infects the area scratched and the wound refuses to heal normally. One to two weeks later, the area may still be red and pus is present. One to six weeks after the scratch, the child's lymph nodes begin to swell and become tender and red. The child will develop a low-grade fever (under 100° F). There may be a loss of appetite, general achiness, and discomfort.

As the disease progresses, the lymph nodes may drain spontaneously and discharge pus through the skin. Complications of cat scratch disease can include Parinaud's oculoglandular syndrome, encephalitis, and granulomas of the liver and spleen. There are approximately 22,000 cases of this disease reported each year, but because of the general nature of the symptoms, many more mild cases may go untreated.

NATURAL CHOICES
Carefully supervise any young child around animals. Don't allow them to pick up or hold cats or kittens unless an adult is present.

For all cat bites or scratches, it is important to clean the area carefully. Wash the area with an antibacterial soap, like Dial, for at least ten minutes.

OVER-THE-COUNTER PRODUCTS

When the wound has been cleaned thoroughly, apply a topical skin antibiotic, like Neosporin (neomycin, polymyxin B, bacitracin), twice a day. Watch the area carefully for signs of redness and pus, possibly indicating an infection.

Pain relievers and fever reducers, like Tylenol (acetaminophen) or Motrin (ibuprofen), may help keep the fever down and make the child more comfortable.

DOCTOR VISITS

If cat scratch disease is suspected, the doctor may do a blood test. He is looking for IgG and IgM antibodies against the *Bartonella henselae* bacteria. If these are present, then it is a positive sign your child is infected.

For most cases, the disease resolves on its own without treatment. However, antibiotics, like Zithromax (azithromycin), Bactrim (sulfamethoxazole/trimethoprim), and erythromycin, may be prescribed to speed recovery. For more serious cases, a course of the intravenous antibiotic gentamycin may be given. If the lymph nodes break down, surgical drainage and removal may be required.

CHICKEN POX

Chicken pox is a highly contagious illness caused by a virus from the herpes family called varicella. It is more common in children under the age of nine, but may occur at any age. The virus spreads by entering through the nose after an infected person sneezes, coughs, or shares food or drinks. Chicken pox can also be spread when the virus gets on little hands that aren't washed before touching the mouth or face or can spread from skin-to-skin contact when open sores develop. A person infected with chicken pox can spread the virus before they develop any symptoms. Pregnant women, newborn infants, and young adults 15 years and older are more likely to have a severe case of chicken pox and develop complications from the infection than young children.

The first symptoms are usually a low-grade fever, accompanied by the child feeling grumpier than normal. Within the next few hours, the face and head will be covered with a red rash. The red rash develops liquid-filled blisters on top. It's when these blisters break open that intense itching begins. This process continues over the next seven to ten days. The chicken pox vaccine is recommended for children and adults who haven't had the disease.

NATURAL CHOICES
There are a few things to do if your child becomes infected with chicken pox:

- Encourage your child not to scratch the bumps as she may increase the risk of permanent scars. Trim your child's fingernails short before the scratching starts, which can help keep those scars to a minimum.

■ Apply wet compresses of baking soda directly to the skin to provide quick relief.

■ Have your child take a bath of cool water with baking soda added which can be wonderful for itchy skin. Also add a cupful of uncooked oatmeal, which will soothe and cool the blisters.

■ As your child may not have much of an appetite during this ordeal, consider allowing them to eat their favorite foods, like ice cream, even if it normally isn't on the preferred menu.

OVER-THE-COUNTER PRODUCTS

For pain relief and fever reduction, Tylenol (acetaminophen) or Motrin (ibuprofen) are good choices. Remember that this is one of the diseases to especially avoid giving your child aspirin. Reye's syndrome (see Reye's Syndrome, pg. 282) has been linked to chicken pox and the use of aspirin.

Oatmeal baths, like Aveeno, help soothe hot skin and ease the itch. Aveeno also makes a cream form for intense itching. Antihistamines, like Benadryl (diphenhydramine), help control the itch from the inside. Calamine lotion is wonderful as a drying agent when the blisters begin to weep. Caladryl lotion combines the drying agent of calamine lotion with the topical anti-itch of Benadryl. It does double duty. Keeping the bottle cool is a nice trick for even more relief.

DOCTOR VISITS

If your child has a serious medical condition that could weaken his immune system, the doctor may prescribe the antiviral medicine Zovirax (acyclovir). To be effective, it must be given within the first 24 hours of first seeing the rash. By the time the bumps appear, it's often too late for antiviral medicines to work.

COLD SORES AND FEVER BLISTERS

These terms cause a great deal of confusion among pharmacy shoppers. Parents ask, "Does my child have a cold sore or fever blister?" The answer is, both. Cold sores and fever blisters are the same condition, and the names are often used synonymously. For the ease of simplicity, we'll refer to them as cold sores.

A cold sore starts out as clusters of small blisters on the lip and outer edge of the mouth. The skin around the blisters is often red and inflamed. After a few days, the blisters break open and the cold sore gets a dry, crusty top. Although cold sores may be unsightly, they aren't typically very painful.

The cause of a cold sore is the herpes simplex virus Type 1, not a fever or cold as their name suggests. The virus may be coaxed out of dormancy by a fever, a cold, or a sunburn on the face. Cold sores are very contagious, and it is estimated that the virus at one time or another has infected nearly half of the population. Once your child develops a cold sore, he should be prepared for frequent recurrence because the virus does not go away but stays dormant in the body until triggered again.

NATURAL CHOICES
It's rare, but the first episode of cold sores can be so painful that your child may have difficulty eating, drinking, and sleeping. Fluids and soft foods, like ice cream or gelatin, can help them get through the worst of the pain.

At the first sign of a cold sore tingling sensation, place an ice cube in a plastic bag and keep the cold area on your child's sore for about five minutes every two to three hours. Studies have shown that the virus can't thrive in a cold environment and that your child may avoid the outbreak entirely.

OVER-THE-COUNTER PRODUCTS

Zilactin Cold Sore Gel has benzyl alcohol as an active ingredient. It forms a protective film over the cold sore to help reduce the pain of eating, drinking, and talking. This product can be used by children over the age of two with adult supervision. It should be applied three to four times daily; relief is usually seen for six hours.

For children over the age of 12, one of the hottest products on the market is Abreva (docosanol). It treats cold sores on the face or lips. It also shortens the healing time and duration of cold sore symptoms, including tingling, pain, burning, and itching. For the best results, start the treatment at the first sign of a tingling sensation and apply up to five times daily until the cold sore is gone.

DOCTOR VISITS

Cold sores may break open and allow a bacterial infection to take hold. If you notice unusual redness around the sore or it appears to be spreading, a prescription antibacterial cream, like Bactroban (mupirocin), may be prescribed.

Older children may benefit from the antiviral cream Denavir (penciclovir). This is used directly on the cold sore every two hours while awake for a total of four days.

COLDS

Children's colds are a common occurrence. In fact, American children miss 23 to 26 million school days each year because of colds! The runny nose, sore throat, coughing, stuffiness, low-grade fever (under 101° F), and sneezes all are part of the joy of a common cold. Colds are caused by a type of virus, called the rhinovirus because of its affinity for the nose.

The virus is spread through direct contact, by, for example, little hands touching their nose, their friends, and, of course, their caregivers. It takes generally 24 to 72 hours from the time of exposure to the first appearance of symptoms, and the child is contagious before the symptoms appear, as well as shortly after all the symptoms have disappeared.

A typical cold lasts about a week, but some children seem to just get over one when they bring home another. With a cold, treatment relies on taking care of the symptoms, as the virus must simply run its course. That can be a confusing task as you comb through the multitude of children's cold products on the pharmacy shelf.

NATURAL CHOICES
Because colds are transmitted by direct contact, the best way to prevent colds from coming home is to stop the virus from being passed around. Here are some tips that may help:

■ Teach your child to use disposable tissues to wipe his runny nose rather than using his sleeve or hands.

■ Emphasize proper hand-washing after coughs and sneezes.

- Wash the toys of a sick child with an antibacterial solution.

- Have your child avoid other sick children if at all possible.

Cool mist humidifiers are wonderful for soothing irritated airways and easing congestion. They use water at room temperature and push it through a rotating disk to form tiny water droplets. They should be cleaned after every use with a bleach or alcohol mixture to kill bacteria, viruses, or fungi that find a home there.

Steam vaporizers allow medicinal additives, like Vicks Vapo-Steam, to be added to the machine for extra cough and congestion-fighting power. Use care with this type of vaporizer due to potential for burns from hot steam.

OVER-THE-COUNTER PRODUCTS

For safe congestion relief in babies as young as three months, try Johnson's Soothing Vapor Bath. It has a wonderful combination of eucalyptus, menthol, and rosemary oils to relax a fussy little one and help them breathe better.

Due to the variety of symptoms your child may have with a cold, it is usually helpful to pick products to fit her specific needs. Using any over-the-counter cough and cold medicine is not recommended for infants under nine months unless given specific instructions from the doctor. Read the package instructions carefully before giving any over-the-counter medicine to your child. Here are some specific product suggestions:

- **Coughs:** Robitussin-DM syrup or Infant Drops

- **Sore throats:** Dimetapp "Get Better Bear" Freezer Pop

- **Fever and aches:** Children's or Infant's Tylenol or Motrin

■ **Nasal decongestants:** Otrivin Pediatric Nasal Drops

■ **Antihistamines:** Benadryl Allergy Liquid

DOCTOR VISITS

Doctor visits aren't required for colds unless the child has a secondary infection, like an earache (see Earache, pg. 207) or pink eye (see Pink Eye, pg. 274). Antibiotics are ineffective against the cold virus. If the fever is higher than 101.3° or lasts more than two days, or if the cold itself hangs around for more than two weeks, then give the doctor a call.

COLIC

Colic is defined as the extreme end of normal crying behavior in a baby from three weeks to five months of age. A determination of colic versus regular crying is made when the baby cries for more than three hours a day, more than three days a week. These long periods of fussiness and piercing cries affect ten to 20 percent of all babies. There is no diarrhea, throwing up, abdominal pain, or fever with colic. Only in five percent of cases was a specific source found to be causing the irritability and forceful crying.

Because crying is such a basic part of an infant's development, it is often difficult to distinguish colic from regular developmental crying. During a colic episode, the baby cries loudly and continuously, may have a red face and clenched fists, arches his back, and holds a hard, tight stomach. The legs may pull up tight to the tummy. The baby generally refuses to be comforted, but is otherwise healthy and well-fed.

As the cause of colic is thought to be an inability of the infant to process nervous stimulation and regulate his crying response, as his system matures, the crying becomes more controlled and easily managed. Therefore, even though the frequency and duration of screaming is tough, it's important to realize that once the doctor diagnoses colic, this is something that your baby will outgrow. Most outgrow it completely by the age of five to six months.

NATURAL CHOICES

Babies with colic are often highly sensitive to their environment. If your baby has colic, limit excess stimulation by keeping her room darkened. Also keep her away from loud noises to better help her focus her sensory perception.

Apply a warmed cloth over a cloth diaper on your child's tummy, which may soothe the fussy crying.

If colic isn't a certainty, rule out other causes by doing the following:

- Check for wet diapers, diaper rash, diarrhea, constipation, something hurting the child, or trapped arms or legs.

- Check for fever, runny nose, sores, or a lump in the groin area (hernia).

- Check for hunger by offering a feeding. Carefully burp during and after each feeding.

OVER-THE-COUNTER PRODUCTS

Because colic is a developmental problem rather than an actual condition, over-the-counter products won't have much effect to calm the crying.

DOCTOR VISITS

It is very important to take the little one in to the doctor if you suspect colic. Unfortunately, infants can't tell us exactly what's making them so miserable. There could be many reasons for the intense crying, and your pediatrician will want to rule each one out.

The baby's formula may be changed in case there is a problem with digestion or a blood and urine test may be run to rule out other problems, but for the majority of cases, colic is rarely tied to a specific cause.

CONGESTION

Your little one wakes up with a stuffy nose. As the day progresses, she can't breathe through her nose at all. She doesn't seem uncomfortable, but you worry about naptime and how the family will sleep through the night.

Her stuffed nose is likely caused by a cold or a seasonal allergy. Allergens, like pollen, pet dander, or mold find a home in the nose, and the body produces histamines to fight the foreign invaders. Nasal passages swell and it becomes difficult to breathe through the nose. Colds, accompanied by the obligatory stuffy nose, are a common occurrance in most children throughout the year.

NATURAL CHOICES

Increasing fluids, like water or juice, can help thin mucus from nasal secretions and reduce congestion. Adding 50 percent water to fruit juice is one way to cut the sugar content. Caffeine-containing sodas and teas should be avoided because it can dehydrate the child. Milk or milk products may increase mucus production, so take a break from these until your child is breathing easier.

For young children, prop the head up with extra pillows at night to promote drainage and decrease congestion. Cool mist humidifiers are wonderful for soothing irritated airways and easing congestion. They use water at room temperature and push it through a rotating disk to form tiny water droplets. They should be cleaned after every use with a bleach or alcohol mixture to kill bacteria, viruses, or fungi that find a home there.

Steam vaporizers allow medicinal additives, like Vicks Vapo-Steam, to be added to the machine for extra cough and congestion-fighting power. Use care with this type of vaporizer due to potential for burns from hot steam.

OVER-THE-COUNTER PRODUCTS

Over-the-counter choices for a child who is congested include decongestants and antihistamines. Decongestants specifically focus on un-stuffing the child, while antihistamines help decrease the body's allergic response to allergens.

Decongestants come in oral (taken by mouth) and nasal (taken through the nose) forms. They decrease swelling in the blood vessels lining the nosal passages and reduce congestion. Decongestants also help to drain the Eustachian tubes in the ears. This type of drainage helps prevent ear infections.

Most oral forms of decongestant have pseudoephedrine as the active ingredient. Be on the lookout for restlessness and insomnia with oral forms.

Those decongestants given through the nose, as drops or sprays, work faster and have fewer nervous side effects. Brands to look for are Otrivin Pediatric Nasal Drops and Afrin Nasal Decongestant Children's Mist. However, nose drops and sprays should only be used for a maximum of three to five days due to the potential for rebound congestion.

For the child who doesn't like the feel of medicinal nose drops, or for the younger set, saline drops, gels, or sprays (like Nasal) are a good choice.

Newer over-the-counter antihistamines, like Claritin (loratidine), often are used to decrease allergy symptoms for children over the age of six. Claritin is available in quick-dissolving RediTabs and pleasant-tasting liquids. The older over-the-counter products, like Benadryl (diphenhydramine), may cause either extreme excitement or drowsiness in children and it's often hard to predict the response. Check with the doctor for a specific antihistamine recommendation for your child.

DOCTOR VISITS

Seldom does ordinary congestion require a trip to the doctor's office. Even nasal discharge with a thick, green color is not recommended for treatment with antibiotics unless it lasts for more than two weeks.

Some of the newer nonsedating antihistamines are still available only by prescription, such as Zyrtec and Allegra, and your child's doctor may want to try these.

CONSTIPATION

Constipation is the passage of large and painful stools or going four or more days without a bowel movement. Children's bowel habits are different from adults. As long as a child is passing soft stools at least every three to four days, constipation is not considered to be a diagnosis.

Constipation occurs when the large intestine absorbs too much water from food waste and the stool becomes hard and difficult to pass. A stool that appears twice the normal diameter is too hard to pass comfortably. The child may hold in her stools in anticipation of discomfort, and this creates a difficult cycle to break.

Most causes of constipation can be traced to these factors:

■ A diet with too much milk (more than 12 to 16 ounces per day).

■ A diet with too little fiber.

■ Waiting too long to empty the bowels.

■ Not drinking enough water.

NATURAL CHOICES

Constipation can usually be effectively taken care of at home with a few dietary modifications. The goal is one to two soft stools each day, but the frequency isn't as important as the consistency.

■ **Increase fluids.** For infants, give two to four ounces of water or a 75/25 mixture of water and apple, pear or prune juice. For older children, increase liquids to a minimum of two to three glasses per day. Avoid milk as a liquid choice, as this increases constipation.

■ **Increase fiber.** Baby foods, like cooked peas, apricots, prunes, peaches, plums, and spinach, are good for the younger set. Fresh fruits and vegetables, like beans, sweet potatoes, corn, and raw tomatoes, along with vegetable soups, help move things along for older children.

■ **Limit constipating foods.** The list includes cow's milk, cheese, yogurt, bananas, and cooked carrots.

OVER-THE-COUNTER PRODUCTS

Home treatment of constipation is not recommended for children under the age of two years. Stimulant laxatives or enemas should not be used on children unless specifically requested by the pediatrician.

Over-the-counter medications for constipation commonly recommended by doctors include stool softeners, like Colace Syrup (docusate sodium), or gentle laxatives, like Metamucil or Milk of Magnesia (MOM). MOM even has a chocolate cream flavor the kids don't mind taking as much. These laxatives make stools easier to pass, but don't cause the stomach cramping associated with stimulant laxatives.

Glycerin suppositories are often effective for bringing on fast constipation relief. Fleet Babylax Liquid Glycerin Suppositories are a gentle, safe way to relieve your child's discomfort from constipation for ages two to five years. These are used rectally and the instructions are "just insert, squeeze, remove, and throw away." It takes just seconds to use and works in 15 minutes to one hour.

DOCTOR VISITS

For constipation concerns, a visit to the doctor is in order if:

■ Constipation or changes in the stool continue for 24 hours in a baby younger than three months.

■ The older child's constipation lingers for one week, even after home treatment has been tried.

■ Pain develops in the rectum or lasts longer than one week.

■ Abdominal pain develops.

■ Blood appears in the stool.

■ Constipation becomes more frequent or more severe.

Prescription medications to relieve constipation include Lactulose syrup and Miralax powder.

COUGH

A cough is the body's natural reflex to clear something from the airway. A cough isn't a condition, but a symptom of something else going on in the body. There are two types of coughs: the wet, or productive cough cough that brings up sputum and the dry, hacking nonproductive cough, where nothing is brought up.

For children, a cough can signal a more serious problem brewing, especially if he is having difficulty breathing. Asthma, pneumonia, bronchitis, and croup are all respiratory conditions where coughing is a symptom. The doctor should check out a persistent cough that is causing any child to have trouble sleeping, is accompanied by a fever, or is interfering with daily activities.

NATURAL CHOICES

Cool mist humidifiers are wonderful for soothing irritated airways and easing coughs. They use water at room temperature and push it through a rotating disk to form tiny water droplets. They should be cleaned after every use with a bleach or alcohol mixture to kill bacteria, viruses, or fungi that find a home there.

Steam vaporizers allow medicinal additives, like Vicks Vapo-Steam, to be added to the machine for extra cough and congestion-fighting power. Use care with this type of vaporizer due to potential for burns from hot steam.

Eliminating the child's exposure to cigarette or pipe smoke or other irritants is effective for easing some types of coughs.

Water acts as a natural expectorant, thinning mucus secretions and making coughs more productive. Adding lots of fluids is a good idea with any cough. Avoid milk during the course of a cold if possible, as milk and milk products may increase sticky mucus production and make it harder for your child to breathe.

OVER-THE-COUNTER PRODUCTS

Over-the-counter cough preparations come in many confusing types. These products aren't recommended for children under the age of two unless specifically requested by the pediatrician. Also, because a cough is a symptom, rather than a disease itself, ask the doctor before using over-the-counter cough suppressants or expectorants. If the doctor gives the okay, here is a breakdown of what to look for on the shelves:

■ **Cough suppressants.** These are to be used when the cough interferes with sleeping or daily activities. Children with asthma or pneumonia should not be taking medicines to suppress a cough. Robitussin-DM Syrup or Robitussin Infant Drops both contain the cough suppressant dextromethorphan. For 12-hour dosing, Delsym (dextromethorphan) is a good choice.

■ **Expectorants.** These loosen mucus, thin bronchial secretions, and make it easier to cough up sticky mucus. Guaifenesin is found in regular Robitussin—the one without any DMs, CFs, or PEs after the name. Each initial after the name means there are other ingredients in the medicine that your child may not need.

DOCTOR VISITS

For tough coughs that don't respond to home treatments, the doctor may write a prescription for a cough syrup containing codeine. Codeine controls coughs by suppressing the cough center in the brain.

If your child is coughing up sputum with a yellowish, green, or brown appearance, there may be a bacterial infection present. A sample will be taken, and if there are bacteria and white blood cells, an antibiotic will be prescribed.

CRADLE CAP

Cradle cap, also called seborrheic dermatitis, is an oily, yellow crusting on an infant's scalp. It is caused by a buildup of sticky skin oils and sloughed skin cells. Cradle cap typically occurs in the "soft spot" area of the scalp and resembles a thick, scaly cap. Cradle cap symptoms seem to run in families. Experts seem to think cradle cap is caused by hormones passed on to the baby from its mother. Those hormones stimulate the oil-producing glands in the baby's scalp and create the problem.

A common worry among parents is that the condition may be contagious. It is not. Nor is cradle cap caused by an allergy or poor hygiene, although fear of cleaning the delicate area can contribute to the problem. Seborrheic dermatitis is simply a skin condition a baby will likely outgrow. It generally disappears by the time the child is eight months old. However, there are cases of cradle cap occurring in children through the age of five.

NATURAL CHOICES

Treatment at home is usually all that is needed for cradle cap. Try these steps to take care of the yellow skin plaques:

■ Before shampooing, rub your baby's scalp with baby oil, mineral oil, or petroleum jelly to help lift the crusts and loosen plaques.

■ When ready to shampoo, first get the scalp wet, then gently scrub the scalp with a soft-bristled brush (a soft toothbrush works well) for a few minutes to remove the scales. You can also try gently removing the scales with a fine-tooth comb or soft sponge.

■ Wash the scalp well, but gently, with a mild shampoo specifically for babies, like Johnson's Baby Shampoo or Pure Baby Cradle Cap Shampoo with Biotin and Vitamin E. Rinse well, and gently towel dry.

OVER-THE COUNTER PRODUCTS

Check with the pediatrician first, but some doctors will advise using a topical over-the-counter steroid cream, like hydrocortisone, to decrease the inflammation and spread of the rash. For areas with open sores from itching, a topical antibiotic, like Bacitracin, may be advised by the doctor. Some doctors also recommend over-the-counter dandruff shampoos for a baby's scalp. Talk to your child's doctor before using a dandruff shampoo, such as Selsun Blue, Head and Shoulders, or Sebulex. If these products get in the baby's eyes, they can cause irritation. Always check with the baby's doctor before putting any over-the-counter product on their scalp, as medications are easily absorbed through thin skin.

Pure Baby Cradle Cap Care with Vitamins A and E in a sensitive skin formula used twice monthly may help prevent a recurrence of cradle cap in susceptible infants.

DOCTOR VISITS
If cradle cap spreads or begins to look red and irritated, call the pediatrician. A stronger steroid cream may be prescribed. In severe cases, shampoos containing coal tar or salicylic acid are often prescribed for daily use until the problem clears up.

CROUP

A child with the croup will often sound much worse than his condition really is. Croup is an infection and swelling of the windpipe, throat, and lower airways. It is caused by a virus and forces a barking cough, hoarseness, and difficulty breathing in. The cough has been compared to that of a barking seal and the sound of breathing in to that of a high-pitched crow.

This contagious infection is seen in children from six months to seven years old. The virus is spread from airborne droplets or by having direct contact with an infected child. It is more common in the late fall and early winter and generally only lasts two to five days. The croup usually seems better during the day, but worsens at night.

Croup begins like a typical cold, with a runny nose and slight cough, and then progresses rapidly into the distinctive cough. Only a slight fever occurs with croup, but the loud, barking cough and whistling or crowing sounds the child makes when breathing in and out cause more alarm among adults than to the child. Croup can become serious very quickly when the airway swells and shuts off incoming air. Keeping a close eye on the child during a croup infection can avoid complications.

NATURAL CHOICES

For mild cases of the croup, home treatment is all that is needed. Encourage lots of fluids and lots of rest. Playing hard and becoming excited can make breathing more difficult.

Cool mist humidifiers are wonderful for soothing irritated airways and easing congestion. They use water at room temperature and push it through a rotating disk to form tiny water droplets. Allow the cool air to blow directly on your child's face.

If this doesn't open the blocked airways, then try warm steam treatment. Bring your child into a small bathroom and turn on hot water faucets to create a moist steam room. Hold your child quietly in your lap as they breathe in the air. This may take 15 to 20 minutes to become effective.

OVER-THE-COUNTER PRODUCTS

Over-the-counter decongestants, antihistamines, or cough/cold products aren't recommended for the treatment of croup. If your child has a fever, Tylenol (acetaminophen) or Motrin (ibuprofen) may be used to control the fever and make him more comfortable.

DOCTOR VISITS

If your child's breathing becomes labored and it is difficult for him to bring in air, head to the doctor's right away. If swelling blocks the airway, call 911 immediately. Look for a rapid heart rate, bluish skin discoloration, flaring of the nostrils, tiredness, or dehydration as symptoms requiring immediate medical attention.

Oxygen may be given in the hospital, as well as medications like epinephrine that quickly open the airways to allow easier breathing. Oral steroids, like dexamethasone or prednisolone, decrease swelling and inflammation rapidly.

DEHYDRATION

There are many ways a child can become dehydrated. Throwing up, diarrhea, diabetes, and excessive sweating are common causes for this potentially dangerous condition. When more fluids are lost from small bodies than are taken in, normal body functions are at risk. The brain, heart, kidneys, and all other body systems depend on a specific combination of fluid electrolytes to function properly.

Important minerals, salts, and water normally present in body fluids are lost quickly in young children. In fact, the younger the child, the more serious dehydration can be. An average of 222,000 children under the age of five are hospitalized each year with complications from dehydration.

NATURAL CHOICES
Prevention is best found by ensuring your child is drinking as much water as possible. One of the first signs of dehydration is a dry mouth or excessive thirst. In most instances, simply drinking more fluids will allow your child's body to correct the imbalance. Allow sips of water with ice chips while they're feeling ill, and provide larger quantities when the weather is warm or your child is playing outside. Weak, decaffeinated teas with sugar, sugar-containing gelatins, fruit juices, and ginger ales are good choices for fluid replacement.

Avoid caffeine-containing drinks, as these can have a diuretic effect, dehydrating your child even more. Milk or milk products should also be avoided.

If excessive sweating is the problem, play or exercise should be moved to a cooler location or suspended until your child's body has a chance to cool down.

OVER-THE-COUNTER PRODUCTS

Electrolyte replacement liquids are a combination of water, sodium (salt), potassium, chloride, and glucose (sugar) that help the body recover from fluid loss by replacing what was lost. These come in a variety of favorite flavors. Putting a bottle in the refrigerator to keep it cold increases the chances that your child will find the flavor acceptable. Brands available from the pharmacy shelf include Pedialyte and Infalyte. Keep in mind that once opened, a bottle is only good for 48 hours before it should be discarded. Pedialyte now has single-serving, half-pint squeeze bottles that are fun and easy to hold. These come in tasty cherry and apple flavors.

As an extra special treat on hot days, try Pedialyte Freezer Pops. These have a long shelf life in the freezer, but be certain to use by the manufacturers' expiration date on the box or throw away. These pops are also an excellent way to keep electrolyte replacement handy in case someone comes down with the stomach flu in the middle of the night. These contain the right mix of sodium (salt), potassium, and glucose (sugar) to replace electrolytes lost from diarrhea and vomiting. An added bonus is that they feel so good on little sore throats.

DOCTOR VISITS

If you suspect dehydration, have your child examined by the doctor right away. If hospitalization is required, intravenous fluids and salts are administered to bring the body fluids back into balance.

Without adequate fluids, the danger of dehydration poses a serious health risk for children. Signs of dehydration to be aware of when your child has diarrhea, is vomiting, or both include:

For infants:

■ Fewer than six wet diapers per day.

■ A sunken soft spot.

■ Skin that has a bread-dough feeling and stays indented when touched or folded.

For toddlers and young children:

■ No tears when crying.

■ Skin that has a bread-dough feeling and stays indented when touched or folded.

■ Dark urine with a strong odor.

■ Inactivity or lethargy.

■ Sunken eyes.

■ A dry mouth.

■ Blotchy and cool hands and feet.

■ A fast and weak pulse.

■ No urination for several hours.

If your child has any of the above signs, contact the doctor right away.

DIAPER RASH

Diaper rash is an irritation of the skin in the diaper area. Most cases of diaper rash occur because a child's tender skin comes into contact with his urine or stools. Irritating chemicals, like those in laundry detergents, soaps, powders, or lotions, may cause an allergic reaction closely resembling a diaper rash. These irritants will aggravate an already tender bottom.

Children taking a course of antibiotics are more prone to diarrhea, which in turn makes a child in diapers more likely to develop a diaper rash. Most children will experience at least one bout of diaper rash during their growth. Signs and symptoms of a diaper rash can vary from mild redness with accompanied soreness to painful, open sores in the diaper area.

There are three types of diaper rashes based on what causes the annoying skin complaint:

1. **Friction rashes.** Chafing contact between the diaper and a baby's skin causes friction rashes. These red areas are commonly found along the inner thighs or where the elastic from disposable diapers tends to gather.

2. **Irritant rashes.** Harsh chemicals from laundry detergents, soaps, or lotions cause irritant rashes. Both friction and irritant rashes are characterized by physicians as to how closely they resemble an abstract painting of red splotches.

3. **Intertrigo rashes.** Intertrigo rashes are caused by moist heat, such as when a damp or wet diaper has been left on sensitive skin for too long. Skin appearing red and thin identifies this type of rash.

Wetness of the baby's skin from diaper contents is the common factor in all forms of diaper rash. When the skin in the diaper area is wet, diapers chafe and friction increases. The baby's already thin skin becomes more pliable and easier to tear. Torn skin in combination with stool enzymes, urine, or other irritants causes redness and painful inflammation.

The baby's diaper area may appear red, raw, and cracked. The skin may be painful to the touch or excruciating when urine or stools are exposed to it. Most rashes respond well to treatment and should clear up within three to four days.

NATURAL CHOICES

The best prevention of diaper rash is to keep your baby's bottom as dry as possible. Following are more methods of lowering the risk of a rash:

■ Avoid rubber pants or disposable diapers if a diaper rash is a continual problem.

■ Stay away from strong detergents, bleaches, or lotions.

■ Change diapers frequently and immediately after urination or bowel movements.

■ Wipe your baby's bottom well after changing her diaper, then dry thoroughly. Premoistened towelettes should be avoided on tender, irritated bottoms as they tend to sting and burn. Dye-, alcohol-, and perfume-free wipes are available; however, a soft washcloth dampened with water is often the best choice.

■ After your baby is clean and dry, allow her to go without a diaper covering the irritated area for a half hour between changes. This permits air to circulate around tender skin and speeds healing.

OVER-THE-COUNTER PRODUCTS

Mild, uncomplicated diaper rash can be safely treated at home. Avoid baby oils and baby powders. Oils won't be absorbed well through the skin and can only be completely removed with soap and water. Talc aspirations from baby powders can cause chemical inhalation pneumonia. Over-the-counter anti-fungal products are not recommended for diaper rash.

Look for skin protectants like Desitin or Diaperine (petrolatum ointment or zinc oxide). These agents are spread over the entire area covered by the diaper and form a barrier against urine and feces. A & D Ointment (petrolatum and lanolin) is another general-purpose skin protectant and soother.

DOCTOR VISITS

A rash on the bottom may be the signal that something else is going on. A call to the doctor is in order if any of the following occur:

- The rash persists for more than four days and any home treatments seem to worsen the rash.

- The rash continues to appear bright red or raw-looking for several days despite treatment.

- Small red dots appear on the baby's bottom, which may indicate a fungal infection.

- Large, crusting blisters or pus appear in the rash.

- Your baby develops a fever.

Yeast-like fungal infections of the diaper area are quite common. The fungus *Candida albicans* finds a nice home in the warm, moist areas under the diaper. Broken skin and violent cries when passing urine or stools are signs of *Candida*. When this occurs, prescription treatment is necessary.

The doctor may prescribe Mycostatin (nystatin). This medicine is in a yellowish powder that is applied directly to the bottom with each diaper change. Some pediatricians prefer a combination cream, like Mycolog II, which contains an antifungal agent (nystatin) and a steroid (triamcinolone) to treat swelling, redness, and itching.

DIARRHEA

Diarrhea is characterized by how loose a child's stool is, not how many times the child goes. It is often a guessing game to determine what is causing the problem and the best way to stop it from occurring.

Typical causes of diarrhea among the younger set are diet, food allergies, bacteria, viruses, or parasites. Children on a course of antibiotics often have problems with diarrhea.

Newborns normally have four to six loose bowel movements a day, and breastfed infants may have more. Loose stools themselves aren't a concern unless the child experiences a decreased appetite, weight loss, is throwing up, or has blood in the stool. Diarrhea may become dangerous if a child begins to lose large amounts of water, as dehydration may become a possibility (see Dehydration, pg. 195).

Each child is different in the amount of liquid in and uniformity of their stools, but there are three different degrees of diarrhea to use as a guide:

1. **Mild:** Three to four stools in 24 hours. The stools are loose and watery, but not particularly abundant.

2. **Moderate:** Five to six stools in 24 hours. The stools are loose, but not watery enough to leak out of a diaper.

3. **Severe:** Seven or more stools in 24 hours. The stools are liquid enough to leak out of a diaper and require a total clothing change.

NATURAL CHOICES

Have your child drink clear liquids to keep her hydrated. Water, tea, and ginger ale are good choices. If she is hungry, give her small amounts of banana, rice (or rice cereal), applesauce, toast, or crackers. This diet is known as BRAT: bananas, rice, applesauce, toast. This diet helps give the stools more form. High-fiber foods, like whole grains and leafy vegetables, should be avoided until the diarrhea has subsided. If diarrhea is a frequent problem you may want to change the diet periodically to rule out certain food allergies (see Food Allergies, pg. 230).

OVER-THE-COUNTER PRODUCTS

For children under the age of three, no form of self-treatment is recommended for diarrhea. A child this age can dehydrate quickly, and prompt medical attention is required for any case of prolonged diarrhea.

For children facing fluid loss from diarrhea or throwing up, the high-electrolyte solutions Pedialyte and Infalyte are an aid to replace lost fluids. Pedialyte comes as a drink and as a tasty freezer pop. Keep in mind the dangers of dehydration and stock up on these before a bout of diarrhea forces a midnight trip to the drugstore.

Antidiarrheal medicines, like Children's Kaopectate, contain the clay-like substance attapulgite as an active ingredient. The attapulgite clay absorbs water from the intestines and helps give the stool more bulk. The bottle lists dosages for children three years and older with instructions to consult a doctor for the correct dose for children under three years old.

Imodium-AD (loperamide) is indicated for children over the age of six years and can often slow down diarrhea with a single dose.

Pepto-Bismol, which contains salicylates (a relative of aspirin), should be avoided for those just getting over the flu or chicken pox due to the risk of Reye's syndrome (see Reye's Syndrome, pg. 282). This medicine is recommended for children over the age of three years unless the child's doctor says otherwise.

DOCTOR VISITS

For any case of diarrhea that concerns you, bring the child in for a doctor visit. Prescription medicines, like Reglan (metaclopromide), can be prescribed to slow down the motion of the digestive system and allow stools more time to form. If your child's problem is caused by a bacteria or parasite, then an antibiotic may be prescribed. In many cases, the doctor may simply advise you to wait it out and let the problem run its course. Adult antidiarrhea medicines should be avoided in children.

DIZZINESS

There are a variety of causes for dizziness or vertigo in children. One of the most common is a viral infection of the inner ear, called labyrinthitis, which disturbs the body's normal balance mechanisms. Bacterial ear infections (see Earache, pg. 207) can also cause a child to feel unsteady and woozy. Dizziness may be the symptom of something else going on in the body, such as a fever, headache, or sore throat. Low blood levels of iron (see Anemia, pg. 141) or a low blood sugar level, such as when a meal is missed, can make a child feel shaky. A hot, stuffy, crowded environment and a stressful situation with accompanying anxiety may cause a feeling of dizziness in a child. More serious causes can include anemia, infection, and epilepsy.

Dizziness is rather an abstract concept for a small child. A child under seven years of age suffering dizziness very often reports a headache. The child may also complain that they feel faint, that the room is spinning, or that they feel wobbly or unsteady. They may also feel nauseous or actually be sick. They may become pale, sweaty, or shaky. Caregivers are the best judge of how a very young child's motor skills change. Observe carefully if dizziness is suspected.

NATURAL CHOICES

In most cases, dizziness is not a sign of major illness. It should disappear when the child is given food and allowed to sit down in the fresh air. Encourage liquids and rest if overexcitement may be the cause.

If you suspect the dizziness may be the result of anemia, ensure your child eats a balanced diet. For children who don't get the proper nutrition from their foods, PediaSure may be a good choice. PediaSure is a liquid source of complete, balanced nutrition for children one to ten years of age. It may be used as a nutritional supplement (one to three cans per day) with or between meals.

OVER-THE-COUNTER PRODUCTS

If your child has a viral infection, they can be given Tylenol (acetaminophen) or Motrin (ibuprofen) to bring down fever and make them more comfortable.

DOCTOR VISITS

If your child's dizziness continues without an obvious cause, get medical advice right away. Your child's doctor will recommend treatment for an existing disease or disorder, like an ear infection, that may be causing or contributing to your child's dizziness. If the child loses consciousness, if their breathing seems slow or irregular, or if their dizziness leads to a seizure with twitching of the limbs, call the doctor or 911 for immediate help.

DRUG ALLERGIES

Many parents confuse true drug allergies and drug sensitivities. If your child experiences a reaction to medicine with diarrhea and an upset stomach, but without a rash or swelling or a trip to the emergency room, that usually means a drug sensitivity has occurred. True drug allergies are much more serious.

In the case of both a drug allergy and a drug sensitivity, your child's body reacts violently to something given to make him better. The initial symptoms of a drug allergy may begin with an itchy rash soon after taking the medicine. Within a few minutes several things may begin to happen within the child's body: the body temperature increases quickly with accompanying skin redness (flushing), there is a rapid swelling of the tissues in the throat that may close the airway, the child's breathing may become labored, and the child may experience a drop in blood pressure. The tongue and throat can swell to the point that it is impossible to swallow or breathe. This is called an anaphylactic reaction or anaphylactic shock (see Anaphylactic Shock, pg. 138). Drug allergies can become life threatening if medical attention is not reached immediately.

Drug allergies can be hard to predict because your child may have symptoms of a full allergic reaction even if he previously has taken the drug with no problems. Any drug has the ability to cause an allergic reaction, but typically the penicillin family is to blame. Amoxicillin is a relative of penicillin. Other related drugs are ampicillin, Augmentin, and dicloxacillin. Other drugs commonly seen to cause allergic reactions include sulfa (Bactrim/Septra), phenytoin (Dilantin), insulin, some vaccines, and the contrast dyes used for X rays.

NATURAL CHOICES

For the treatment of drug allergies, the number one choice is avoiding the drug that causes the problem. Inform your child's doctor, dentist, and pharmacist of any problems he has had with medicines in the past. This will help prevent a medicine being prescribed or dispensed for him that could cause an allergic reaction.

OVER-THE-COUNTER PRODUCTS

For mild reactions, antihistamines, like diphenhydramine, taken by mouth or used in cream form can help the itchy hives. Once the drug causing the allergy or sensitivity has been stopped, the hives and other symptoms generally go away on their own within a few days to a week.

DOCTOR VISITS

With an allergic drug reaction, time is very important. If you have recently given your child a medicine and you feel that he is experiencing an allergic reaction, don't waste time. Call 911 or head to the doctor right away. If it is only a mild reaction, the doctor will probably send you on your way with an over-the-counter antihistamine like Benadryl (diphenhydramine) and instructions on what to do should this reaction occur again.

If the allergic reaction appears to be more serious, an epinephrine shot will be administered. The doctor may also write a prescription for a corticosteroid, like prednisolone, to help bring down the swelling in the tissues and help your child breathe better.

If your child's reaction to a particular drug has resulted in swelling and difficulty breathing, it is important to ask the doctor about an anaphylaxis kit, like EpiPen or EpiPen Jr., for future emergencies. These kits are easy to carry in a backpack or purse and contain a shot of epinephrine that just might save your child's life if he accidentally comes into contact again with something that his body is extremely allergic to. Have one for home and one for travel to ensure that medicine is always close by.

If your child has a history of drug allergies that could be life threatening, it is a very good idea to be sure they wear a MedicAlert necklace or bracelet at all times.

EARACHE

With children, earaches generally come on quickly. The first symptoms of an earache are often pain, fever, a slight loss of hearing, and increased fussiness. With infants, detecting an ear infection is a little trickier. Tugging on the ears or shaking the head from side to side are common signs of ear pain in infants.

There may be several reasons for a child to complain of pain in the ear. Otitis media, or infection of the middle ear, is a common problem in children under six years old. In fact, over 80 percent of children will have had at least one middle ear infection by the age of three. With an earache, the pain results from a blockage of the Eustachian tube, which is the canal that drains from the ear to the back of the throat. This tube can become swollen and get plugged up when an infection finds a home in the warm, moist environment of the ear canal.

Children get more earaches than adults because they have narrower tubes than adults do. Weaker immune systems allow them increased susceptibility to colds and respiratory infections. Babies who are bottle fed lying down can develop earaches from milk entering the Eustachian tubes. All of these factors make babies and young children prime targets for ear infections.

Earaches in older children may be attributed to accumulated earwax, improper use of materials to clean the ears, or water accumulation in the ear during swimming or taking showers. Children who spend lots of time at the swimming pool or those who shower frequently can unknowingly strip the normal lining of the ear canal and allow bacterial or fungal growth in the trapped water pockets. If water gets deep into the ear canal and becomes trapped, either by wax accumulation or swelling of the Eustachian tubes, a condition called otitis externa or "swimmer's ear" develops.

Symptoms are itching, pain, draining, persistent ringing, or sloshing in the ear (see Swimmer's Ear, pg. 298).

With proper medical attention, an earache usually clears up in ten to 14 days, but if the fluid in the middle ear gets trapped, there may be lasting problems. Complications of untreated earaches can be serious. It's important to follow up with proper medical attention on an earache, because if the inflammation and fluid buildup continues, the eardrum may be damaged. Long-term hearing loss and delayed communication ability may result for the child if the infection goes on too long.

NATURAL CHOICES

Temporary relief from earaches can often be found by applying warm cloths to the painful ear. Heat applied to the ear and neck can be soothing as well as helpful to expand the plugged and painful Eustachian tubes.

Home remedies are often a good place to start with mild cases of swimmer's ear, where the main symptoms are itching and sloshing. Fill a small dropper bottle from your pharmacy with equal parts isopropyl alcohol, hydrogen peroxide, and water. Place two to four drops in the affected ear daily to dry the water and make the ear canal environment inhospitable to bacteria and fungus.

OVER-THE-COUNTER PRODUCTS

For children's earache pain, a first choice is to help unplug the clogged Eustachian tubes. To accomplish this, try a decongestant like PediaCare Decongestant Drops for Infants or Triaminic Allergy Congestion. Both of these have pseudoephedrine as the active ingredient. The Triaminic products give professional labeling guidelines for younger children based on weight, but, as always, consult your pediatrician or pharmacist if you're unsure of the dosage.

Infant's Tylenol Cold Drops contain both pseudoephedrine as a decongestant and acetaminophen as a fever reducer. These are a good choice for the younger ones with an earache. Many children find some temporary pain relief from Tylenol (acetaminophen) or Motrin oral suspension (ibuprofen) given by mouth.

For older children with swimmer's ear, solutions like Star-Otic and Swim-Ear get into the ear with isopropyl alcohol & anhydrous glycerin to stop the growth of bacteria and fungus, as well as keep the ear canal dry to stop these organisms from returning.

Propylene glycol and Burow's solution ingredients are important as drying agents. Just put three to five drops into the ear canal before and after swimming or bathing, and stop if any irritation occurs.

The Murine Earwax Removal System is good for clearing waxy ears in older children. This product contains the active ingredients anhydrous glycerin and carbamide peroxide. The glycerin softens the wax, while the bubbles released from the carbamide peroxide gently loosen the buildup. Use the bulb syringe provided to flush the ear canal with warm water.

DOCTOR VISITS

Because of the potential for long-term hearing damage, it is important to head for the doctor's office when someone in your family has an earache. The doctor will determine whether the infection is caused by a bacteria or virus. Middle ear infections caused by bacteria are treated with prescription antibiotics.

For bacterial infections, the doctor may prescribe a broad-spectrum antibiotic, like penicillin, Augmentin, or amoxicillin—the liquid we call "the pink stuff." If the dosage of the liquid antibiotic is less than a teaspoonful, ask your pharmacist for a special syringe to make sure the medicine is measured correctly. Antibiotics may be given either alone or in combination with a pain-relieving eardrop, like Auralgan, which has the numbing agent benzocaine to ease the discomfort of a swollen ear canal.

Antibiotic/corticosteroid eardrops, like Cortisporin Otic (neomycin, polymyxin B, and hydrocortisone), penetrate deep into the ear to kill bacteria and relieve inflammation. This is available as both a solution and a suspension.

Some ear infections are caused by a virus, and in cases like this, the doctor may only prescribe an eardrop to ease the pain until the virus runs its course. The eardrops will feel much better going in if you put the capped bottle in a warm cup of water. The warmth will also expand the Eustachian tubes a little, allowing the pain-relieving medication to reach its destination faster.

Getting eardrops into your child's ears can be a daunting task.

Here are some tips for making sure that more medicine gets in the ear rather than all over you and your child:

■ Have your child lie down or tilt her head so the sore ear is facing up.

■ Pull your child's earlobe up and back to give the medicine best access to the Eustachian tube.

■ Place the medicine in your child's ear and allow it to soak in for five minutes.

■ Insert a small wad of cotton into the ear to help keep the medicine deep within the ear canal where it will do the most good.

EARWAX

Earwax, also called cerumen, is the sticky, protective substance inside the ear that catches foreign particles before they have a chance to invade the ear canal.

While not usually a concern, earwax may harden and cause discomfort, dizziness, or ringing in the ears (see Tinnitus, pg. 302). Earaches in older children may also be attributed to accumulated earwax. This wax can build up and trap water deep into the ear canal, where bacteria and fungi find a home. Using objects, like Q-tips or fingers, to try to remove the wax only results in pushing it further against the eardrum. If not removed, the buildup may cause hearing loss. To remove tightly packed earwax, a doctor's visit is in order.

NATURAL CHOICES

While young children may appear to have a great deal of earwax, this is normal. The amount of earwax produced generally decreases as the child gets older and the body matures. The best home course of treatment is to do nothing unless the child complains of discomfort or hearing loss. Earwax is self-draining, and normal amounts will come out on its own. It appears light to dark brown or orange and does not have an unpleasant or foul smell.

If the child's doctor gives permission, try an easy-to-make home earwax softener. Ask your pharmacist for a dropper bottle and add equal parts hydrogen peroxide, mineral oil, and warm water. Use two drops in each ear for one to two days. Warming the entire bottle between your hands for a few minutes will allow the medicine to soften the wax and will feel better going in.

OVER-THE-COUNTER PRODUCTS

For children over the age of 12, there are several commercial products to help soften and remove earwax. However, these should not be used if your child has ear drainage or discharge, ear pain, irritation, a rash in the ear, or dizziness. Also, these should not be used if the child has an injury or perforation in the eardrum, or after ear surgery, unless directed by a physician.

The Bausch and Lomb Ear Wax Removal System contains the active ingredients anhydrous glycerin and carbamide peroxide. Glycerin acts as a wax softener, while the bubbles released from the carbamide peroxide gently loosen the buildup. The bulb syringe provided makes it easy to flush the ear canal with warm water. Debrox also makes a carbamide peroxide drop to place in the ear to soften, loosen, and remove earwax. The Food and Drug Administration has given these products approval as "occasional use" only agents—that is, twice daily for up to four days. If your child's ears are ever painful, please see your doctor. There may be hardened or impacted earwax that has to be removed by the doctor.

DOCTOR VISITS

Some warning signs that earwax may have progressed to the point where prompt medical attention is needed, include:

- Foul-smelling discharge from the ear

- Pain

- Severe itching

- Dizziness

- Fever

- Persistent ringing or fullness in the ear

- Hearing loss

If the wax has hardened and compacted, the best course is to have it removed at the physician's office. The doctor uses a special trumpet-shaped instrument called a speculum. It is placed in the ear canal and a bright light is shined in. The wax is then removed using an instrument called a cerumen spoon.

ECZEMA

With eczema, also called atopic dermatitis, the child's skin becomes very dry, red, itchy, and sensitive. It is a common problem in infants and children, usually appearing between the ages of two and six months. It often starts on the forehead, cheeks, and scalp and spreads to the trunk, creases of the elbows, knees, and wrists. With scratching, the rash may become raw, crusted, and weepy. Infants are especially sensitive to eczema, but normally grow out of it by the age of three.

Eczema conditions run in families; in fact, over 70 percent of cases in children can be directly linked to one or both parents. Eczema also occurs much more frequently in families who already have allergies or asthma. Theories for the cause of this skin condition suggest that the child's body sees the entire outside world as one giant allergen and reacts to it accordingly by breaking out into an itchy rash. Secondary skin infections are a concern because of scratching and the potential for bacteria to find a home in the broken skin. Because your child's body is already busy fighting other invisible foes, these secondary infections can be quite severe.

There is no cure for eczema and there is no one specific cause. The key to treating eczema is to make the symptoms more bearable and the flare-ups less frequent.

NATURAL CHOICES

Help prevent flare-ups by having your child avoid things that are known to trigger his eczema. These may include certain foods, like cow's milk, eggs, peanut butter, and fish; wool fibers and clothes; rough or tight-fitting clothing; dry air; sweating; getting too hot or too cold (including from being exposed to extremely hot or cold water); harsh soaps or chemicals; and stress. Swimming is allowed, but have your child immediately shower or bathe to wash off chlorine and other chemicals. Apply a moisturizer to help prevent your child's skin from drying out.

Also use a lubricating cream, such as Eucerin, Nivea, or Lubriderm, every day, even when the eczema isn't flaring up. Apply these right after baths within three minutes, throughout the day as needed, and after any prescription or over-the-counter eczema creams to help trap in moisture. For severely dry skin, try using an ointment, such as Aquaphor.

Keep your child's fingernails clean and short to limit the skin damage and possible infection caused by scratching.

OVER-THE-COUNTER PRODUCTS

For mild eczema attacks, Benadryl (diphenhydramine) and hydrocortisone creams are effective to control the itching for a short time. Ask your child's doctor when and how much to use. Plain Vaseline petroleum jelly, applied directly to the itchy area, can serve to keep the skin moist and decrease scaling. For nighttime itching, children's diphenhydramine is a good choice to ease the itch from the inside.

Pure Baby Eczema Bath Therapy with biotin and baking soda is specially formulated for your baby's dry, sensitive skin. Eczema Bath Therapy helps soothe, clean, and protect your baby's irritated skin and helps to retain the skin's natural moisture. This product's gentle, nondrying formula is hypoallergenic and 100 percent fragrance and dye free, which pediatricians agree is important in preventing the inflammation of eczema.

DOCTOR VISITS

To determine whether or not your child has eczema, the doctor can do several tests, including the RAST (radioallergosorbent test). If eczema is determined, the typical treatments for flare-ups include steroid creams, like Cutivate or Elocon. Apply these right after a bath, but before a lubricant cream/ointment. Apply again during the day as directed. Be sure to follow the doctor's instructions exactly. These are for short-term use only. Avoid using prescription steroid creams on the face or in the diaper area, unless specifically instructed to do so.

Medications for eczema treatment in children include:

■ Protopic (or tacrolimus), which is an immune system suppressor ointment. It is prescribed in the 0.03 percent strength for the treatment of moderate to severe atopic dermatitis (eczema) for children over the age of two. It is usually prescribed when other therapies have not been effective.

■ Elidel (or pimercrolimus) is another nonsteroidal cream. It is prescribed in the 1 percent strength for the treatment of mild to moderate atopic dermatitis (eczema) in children over two years of age.

ELECTROLYTE IMBALANCE

When your child is throwing up, has prolonged diarrhea, has stomach flu, has stomach virus (gastroenteritis), or is excessively sweating, there are often excessive amounts of fluid lost. This fluid contains a unique combination of electrolytes, including water, salt, potassium, chloride, and sugars. The brain, heart, kidneys, and all other body systems depend on a specific combination of these fluid electrolytes to function properly. When more fluids are lost from small bodies than are taken in, normal body functions are at risk.

Important minerals, salts, and water normally present in body fluids are lost quickly in young children. In fact, the younger the child, the more serious electrolyte imbalance and the accompanying dehydration can be. An average of 222,000 children under the age of five are hospitalized each year with complications from electrolyte imbalance and dehydration.

NATURAL CHOICES

Prevention is best found by ensuring your child is drinking as much water as possible. One of the first signs of dehydration is a dry mouth or excessive thirst. In most instances, simply drinking more fluids will allow your child's body to correct the imbalance. Allow sips of water with ice chips while they're feeling ill and provide larger quantities when the weather is warm or they are playing outside. Weak, noncaffeinated teas with sugar, sugar-containing gelatins, fruit juices, and ginger ales are good choices for fluid replacement. For an at-home electrolyte replacement substitute, mix four ounces of apple or grape juice with six ounces of cool water. Add one teaspoonful of honey and a dash of salt.

If excessive sweating is the problem, move your child's play or exercise to a cooler location or suspend it until your child's body has a chance to cool down.

Avoid caffeine-containing drinks, as these can have a diuretic effect, dehydrating the child even more. Milk or milk products should also be avoided.

OVER-THE-COUNTER PRODUCTS

Electrolyte replacement liquids, which come in a variety of flavors, are a combination of water, sodium, potassium, chloride, and sugars that help the body recover from fluid loss by replacing what was lost. Put the bottle in the refrigerator to keep it cold, which will increase the chances your child will approve of the taste. Brands available from the pharmacy shelf include Pedialyte and Infalyte. Keep in mind that once opened, these products are only good for 48 hours before the entire bottle should be discarded.

As an extra special treat on hot days, try Pedialyte Freezer Pops. They have a long shelf life stored in the freezer or pantry, but as with most over-the-counter products, throw them away after the manufacturer's recommended product expiration date. These freezer pops are also an excellent way to keep electrolyte replacement handy in case someone comes down with the stomach flu in the middle of the night. These contain the right mix of eloctrolytes to replace those lost from diarrhea and vomiting—and they feel so good on sore throats.

DOCTOR VISITS

If you suspect an electrolyte imbalance leading to dehydration, have your child examined by the doctor right away. If hospitalization is required, intravenous fluids and salts are administered to bring body fluids back into balance.

Without adequate fluids, the danger of dehydration poses a serious health risk for children. Following are signs of dehydration to be aware of when your child has diarrhea, is vomiting, or both.

For infants:

■ The child has produced fewer than six wet diapers per day.

■ The child has a sunken soft spot.

■ The child's skin has a soft, "bread-dough" feeling, where a fold of skin remains pinched or indented when touched.

For toddlers and young children:

■ The child does not produce tears when crying.

■ The child's skin has a "bread-dough" feeling, where a fold of skin remains pinched or indented when touched.

■ The child has dark urine with a strong odor.

■ The child is inactive or lethargic.

■ The child has sunken eyes.

- The child has a dry mouth.

- The child has blotchy face and cool hands and feet.

- The child has a fast and weak pulse.

- The child does not urinate for several hours.

FEBRILE SEIZURES

Febrile (or fever) seizures are frightening events for the first-time parent. When the child's temperature begins to creep upward, the brain begins a mini short circuit and a seizure results. During this time, the child may thrash about with stiff muscles and clenched teeth. His eyes may roll back as he loses consciousness. Afterward, he may remain unresponsive for a short time. Normal activity should resume within one hour of the attack.

These fever-related seizures may last from one to 15 minutes, with three minutes being average. They typically occur in children aged six months to six years. As with treatment of all fevers, the goal is to make the child comfortable without concentrating specifically on bringing down the fever (see Fever, pg. 221).

NATURAL CHOICES
When your child is having a seizure, it is important to move objects away from him rather than trying to move him. Don't try to hold your child down or force him in any way. Ease your child to the floor or, if he is small, put him face down in your lap. Turn his head to the

side so saliva and vomit can come out rather than choke him. Note how long the seizure lasts to describe it to the pediatrician. Your child may appear sleepy and groggy after the seizure. This is normal, and sleep in a cool, quiet place should be encouraged.

OVER-THE-COUNTER PRODUCTS

When your little one is running a fever, over-the-counter fever reducers, called antipyretics, can make them feel a little better. Tylenol (acetaminophen) for children over the age of two should be given every four hours. Motrin (ibuprofen) liquid, for children over six months old, should be given at six- to eight-hour intervals not more than four times a day.

DOCTOR VISITS

While it's easy to say that most febrile seizures are completely harmless and don't require a visit to the doctor, when a parent witnesses their child having a one- to 15-minute seizure, the first instinct is to get him to the hospital. It is okay to follow your instincts. However, here are some answers from *Family Practice News* to common questions parents have when bringing their child in for treatment:

■ Could this seizure have been predicted or prevented? In most cases, no. The only factor that can lead to a prediction of a seizure is if both parents or two first-degree relatives have experienced such a seizure. There is a 30 percent chance of a second seizure for the child after the first one has occurred.

■ Would giving over-the-counter fever reducers decrease the risk of a febrile seizure? No. They can help the child feel more comfortable, but they won't prevent a repeat seizure.

■ Will my child's intellectual performance be affected? No.

If the child experiences a headache, stiff neck, or vomiting after a febrile seizure, bring them into the doctor right away.

FEVER

A parent's fear of their child's fever is understandable. Their small bodies heat up at an alarming rate, their actions become lethargic, and they get very quiet—all very unusual activities for a small child. While temperatures can rise very quickly and dangerously when a child is sick, it is important to realize that a fever is a symptom, not an illness itself.

When a child's temperature begins to rise, it is a sign that something is going on inside her body. A fever usually indicates an inflammation or infection has developed. A fever, or higher than normal body temperature, is a sign that the body's immune system is attacking the bacteria or virus causing the inflammation or infection. If we begin to look at a fever as an indicator, rather than a condition, it makes treatment choices clearer. Sometimes the best treatment is to simply do nothing, which is a hard feat for most parents. Experts recommend that fever only be treated if it is over 102° F or when it makes the child uncomfortable.

If the fever is brought down before it has a chance to do its job, the infection could be prolonged. Here are some fever facts to be aware of:

■ Your child's temperature is usually lower in the morning and higher in the evening.

■ A normal temperature for children can be anywhere in the range of 97° F to 100° F.

■ Fever is defined as over 100.4° F in a newborn or over 101° F in an older child.

■ It is important to talk to the doctor if your child's temperature is above 102° F.

■ Febrile seizures can result from high fevers (see Febrile Seizures, pg. 219).

■ Brain damage or death does not normally occur from a high fever alone.

■ Fevers should always be taken seriously in children who are less than three months old, children with immune system problems, and children undergoing cancer treatments.

NATURAL CHOICES

Some pediatricians recommend giving your child a lukewarm sponge bath to make her more comfortable before heading to the over-the-counter aisle for a fever medication. Lukewarm water helps the child by dilating the blood vessels near the skin and cooling the blood.

Fluids should be encouraged to prevent dehydration. Popsicles or Pedialyte freezer pops are a good way to supplement this. A good sign of the appropriate level of hydration is that your child is urinating at least every six to eight hours.

Check with your child's doctor first before treating a fever if it is below 102° F. If the child has a low fever but does not seem to be uncomfortable and is eating well, it may not be necessary to treat the fever with medication or baths. Monitor how the child is feeling and consult the doctor right away if there is any change in behavior.

OVER-THE-COUNTER PRODUCTS

The first step in treating a fever is determining whether the child has an elevated temperature or not. All homes should have a good thermometer (and maybe two, just in case one is dropped by a bleary parent during the middle of the night). Common thermometers include:

■ **Digital thermometers.** These can be used both orally or rectally. These generally work in less than 30 seconds. An audible beep sounds when the temperature is ready. This is important for low-light or "no glasses" situations. This type of thermometer is inexpensive and easy to use.

■ **Ear thermometers.** This type is used by pediatricians and works in two seconds or less. These are the best for ease of use and accuracy. Read the directions carefully as different brands use differing calibration times.

■ **Glass thermometers.** These are the type we used as children. They come in oral or rectal varieties. Due to the fragile nature of glass thermometers, the dangers of mercury, and the inexpensive price of digital, these are becoming harder to find.

■ **Temperature strips.** These are applied on the forehead and give a reading within seconds. They are easy to use, but not very accurate. They are not recommended for use when a precise temperature measurement is needed.

Caregivers may measure temperature rectally (in the rectum), axillary (under the armpit), orally (in the mouth), or tympanically (in

A Drug Lady Reminder

A rectal thermometer is generally recommended for use in children under five years old for the most precise temperature. It is important to remember that a rectal temperature is 0.5° F to 1° F higher than an oral temperature.

the ear). However, these temperatures won't all be the same. Here is a guide for determining the correct temperature for your child.

- The average normal oral temperature is 98.6° F. An oral temperature is 0.5° F to 1° F lower than a rectal or tympanic temperature.

- A rectal temperature is 0.5° F to 1° F higher than an oral temperature.

- A tympanic temperature is 0.5° F to 1° F higher than an oral temperature.

- An axillary temperature is usually 0.5° F to 1° F lower than an oral temperature.

Liquid Tylenol (acetaminophen) is a good first choice for fighting fevers. Available in Infant Drops and Children's Liquid, this product has specific age/weight instructions on the box. Be sure to read them carefully. Aspirin should be avoided to treat fevers in all children under the age of 15 years due to the risk of Reye's syndrome (see Reye's Syndrome, pg. 282).

Another popular choice is Motrin. Liquid Motrin (ibuprofen)

tastes great, works fast, and lasts longer than Tylenol. It's also a great pain reliever because it works as an anti-inflammatory drug as well as a fever reducer. Anti-inflammatory medicines also help bring down the swelling from painful conditions like earaches and teething.

For little ones who can't keep anything down, Feverall (acetaminophen) in the suppository form can be a lifesaver when all else fails. These suppositories must be unwrapped prior to use and are usually very effective for bringing down a fever.

DOCTOR VISITS

Because a fever is the body's way of alerting us that there may be something serious brewing, it is very important to monitor the child carefully for any unusual symptoms or behavior. If you notice that your child is experiencing any of the following symptoms with their fever, call the doctor right away:

- Jerking or shaking motions—which can indicate a seizure.

- Pain—or if mild pain becomes more severe.

- A fever that lasts longer than 72 hours.

- Unusual grogginess or sleepiness.

- A stiff neck or back, confusion, or a spotted rash.

These all may be the first sign of a more serious condition that requires prompt medical attention. Follow your instincts and the thermometer when it comes to your child's fever.

FIFTH DISEASE

The scientific name for Fifth disease is erythma infectiosum. It sounds a bit like something from Harry Potter, doesn't it? This unusual-sounding disease is actually very common among children in the five- to 14-year-old range. Fifth disease got its name from its fifth position in the list of rash-like conditions documented in the early 1900s. It is caused by the human parvovirus B19 and can be easily diagnosed by the "slapped cheeks" appearance of redness on the face.

The early symptoms of the condition are a low-grade fever, aches, chills, and fatigue. Unfortunately, this is the point when the child is contagious and it is often difficult to distinguish this from any number of illnesses. In seven to ten days, the first stage of the rash appears on the cheeks, then the arms, tummy, and legs follow. The rash appears in a lacy pattern. It can come and go for several weeks and is often brought on again by sun exposure, warm baths, or excitement.

For a family member exposed to a child with fifth disease, there is a good chance that they will come down with it also. The disease is spread by close contact. Symptoms appear in one to four weeks after first exposure. Because of the possibility of harm to an unborn child from the virus, pregnant women should avoid contact with an infected person.

NATURAL CHOICES

By the time your child appears with the itchy rash, she is no longer contagious and can attend day care or school without risk to others. However, she is likely to be very uncomfortable and itchy. There are several ways to treat the symptoms of fifth disease and make the child more comfortable:

■ Give your child cool baths and dress them in breathable, non-binding clothes to remedy the itch.

■ Have your child play inside on hot days to reduce the rash and possibly prevent a recurrence.

■ In order to avoid a recurrence of the condition, limit your child's hot baths and showers until the rash has disappeared for several weeks.

OVER-THE-COUNTER PRODUCTS

For the chills, fever, and aches in the early stages of the disease, children's doses of Tylenol (acetaminophen) or Motrin (ibuprofen) are effective.

Old-fashioned calamine lotion is one of the best ways to cool the itch. Today there are brands with the anti-itch ingredient diphenhydramine (Caladryl) as well as clear formulas to avoid the embarrassing pink spots.

DOCTOR VISITS

The doctor will typically rule out any other conditions that may be causing the rash, such as roseola, scarlet fever, or measles. Fifth disease is a self-limiting ailment, which means that it must run its course. There is no specific medical treatment or prevention of fifth disease. If the child has a blood or immune system disorder, hospitalization may be required until the disease has subsided to ensure no complications develop.

The greatest danger of this condition occurs when a pregnant woman is exposed to a child with fifth disease. Warnings for pregnant women exposed to fifth disease are to protect the unborn fetus. Because of the low risk of miscarriage (1.5 percent to 2.5 percent) among women who are infected with the virus, it is important to let the doctor know of possible exposure as soon as possible.

FLU

The flu, or influenza, is a respiratory condition caused by a virus, influenza A or influenza B. This virus is spread from droplets in the air from coughs, sneezes, or sharing saliva with someone who has the virus.

Influenza in children can be a very serious illness. The child is at higher risk for hospital stays, as well as more long-term risks of developing pneumonia, heart problems, ear infections, and croup.

Symptoms of the flu include chills (usually coming on suddenly), a high temperature of 102° F to 106° F (also coming on quickly), sore throat, headache, body aches, redness in the face and eyes, and pain in the joints. There may also be diarrhea and vomiting.

The high fever typically lasts three to five days. It is usually high for the first day or two, normal for a day, then it spikes again for one to two more days. However, the weakness and body aches may continue for one to two weeks. Isolating children with the flu is the best mode of preventing its spread.

NATURAL CHOICES

Bed rest is important, so this could be an opportunity to finish reading that book the two of you started ages ago. Once the initial high fever has passed, the child's immune system may be weakened, so it's best to keep him away from other children to prevent a secondary infection from finding a home.

Children in close proximity to each other in day care or school classrooms are germ magnets. However, by stressing a few tips for both home and school, the spread of bacteria and viruses may be kept to a minimum:

■ Encourage your child to cover his mouth when coughing or sneezing.

■ Encourage your child to wash his hands after every cough, sneeze, or nose wiping.

■ Tell your child not to share cups and utensils with someone who is sick.

■ Have your sick child stay home if possible. The flu virus can be spread for up to ten days after symptoms first appear.

OVER-THE-COUNTER PRODUCTS

If the doctor has diagnosed your child with the flu, there are things you can do to make him more comfortable. Encourage him to drink fluids. Water is best, but high-calorie, high-electrolyte products like Pedialyte help avoid dehydration.

To ease sore throats, the freezer pops from Pedialyte are a good choice. These also help with increasing fluid intake.

Children's pain relievers, like Tylenol (acetaminophen) or Motrin (ibuprofen), are helpful to ease the fever, muscle aches, headache, and chills that often accompany the flu. Be very careful to avoid any products containing aspirin or salicylates during the influenza due to the possibility of Reye's syndrome (see Reye's Syndrome, pg. 282).

DOCTOR VISITS

The best treatment for the flu is prevention. The Centers for Disease Control (CDC) recommends vaccination of healthy children aged six to 23 months due to immature immune systems before the age of two. The CDC also recommends that *all* high-risk children—those with chronic lung problems (like asthma), heart disease, and diabetes—from age six months to 18 years should receive the immunization.

If your child has flu symptoms, bring them to the doctor for a diagnosis and to rule out any other conditions. For children who are susceptible to lung problems or those who may have developed a secondary infection, the doctor may require antibiotics, intravenous fluids, or a hospital visit to ensure no further complications.

FOOD ALLERGIES
(ALSO SEE FOOD ALLERGIES IN HOT TOPICS)

Food allergies and food intolerances are often thought of as being the same thing, when in fact, they are very different. Many parents think their child is allergic to a certain type of food, when in fact, it is only an intolerance to a particular food. In fact, less than two percent of children have genuine food allergies. They are more common in younger children (affecting about five to eight percent of younger children). Fortunately, most younger children will outgrow these food allergies by the time they are three years old.

Food intolerances are different from food allergies. For example, some individuals can't eat dairy products because it upsets their stomach terribly and causes diarrhea. They aren't necessarily allergic to dairy products, but possibly just lack an enzyme called lactase that is necessary to help digest milk and cheese.

A food allergy is characterized by an acute allergic reaction to a particular food. It may also be called serum sickness. With a food allergy, your child's body sees the food as something that must be fought at all costs. Typically, this type of reaction includes rapid swelling of the airways and very itchy hives. It can quickly progress to anaphylactic shock (see Anaphylactic Shock, pg. 138). With swelling of the tongue and throat, it becomes very difficult for the child to breathe. Severe stomach cramps, diarrhea, and nausea may also accompany a food allergy. These types of food allergy symptoms occur with the majority of those cases in children under the age of six.

Foods causing allergic reaction typically include seafood, peanuts, eggs (especially egg whites), milk, soy, wheat, or spinach. "Extras" put into foods, like certain starches or chemicals, can also cause a violent reaction. Look out for corn starch, food dyes (like yellow #5), and gum arabic.

Children with food allergies typically begin showing their allergic reaction with a skin rash. Symptoms may be mild or very severe, depending on how much of the food your child ingested and how allergic she is to the food.

Food-allergic children may also have many more episodes of hay fever and may be more prone to asthma than other children. Some experts speculate on a connection between food allergies, attention deficit disorder, and migraine headaches.

NATURAL CHOICES

Foods to avoid until your infant is at least a year old include cow's milk, citrus fruits and juices, and wheat. Also avoid giving eggs until age two, and peanuts (including smooth peanut butter) and shellfish until your child is at least three years old.

If the child has a true food allergy, the best treatment is to ensure that the child has no further contact with the offending food. There isn't a shot or a pill for your child to take that will enable her to eat the foods she is allergic to. Desensitizing allergy shots are ineffective for food allergies. Once you determine what your child is allergic to, it is important to learn to read food labels because the food your child is allergic to may be an ingredient of many other foods.

If the problem is not a true allergy, but a food sensitivity, like lactose intolerance, then yogurt is a good food choice. For lactose-intolerant children, the bacteria from live yogurt cultures produce *Lactobacillus acidophilus,* an enzyme that is very effective in breaking down lactose. Look for yogurt with "live cultures" listed on the label for the best defense against lactose intolerance (see Lactose Intolerance, pg. 262).

OVER-THE-COUNTER PRODUCTS

Unfortunately, parents of children with true food allergies won't find anything available on the over-the-counter shelves. The best defense is to keep the child away from the food that causes the allergy. However, it is important to be prepared for those instances when you might not be aware that a particular food may cause an allergic reaction. This may happen at times when the little one might sneak "just a tiny bite" of a favorite food or if a commercially prepared food contains an allergy-producing ingredient. It is a good idea for home treatment of hives to have an antihistamine, like diphenhydramine, around for emergencies. For a child with true food allergies, home treatment is not recommended. A prompt doctor's call is in order at the first sign of distress.

DOCTOR VISITS

If the cause of the allergy is uncertain, testing may be done by the doctor. Either skin testing or a RAST, which is a blood test to check for antibodies against certain things your child may be allergic to, may be used to see if specific food allergies can be found.

An anaphylaxis kit, like EpiPen or EpiPen, Jr., is prescribed by the doctor if your child's reaction to a particular food has resulted in swelling and difficulty breathing. These should always be kept on hand for emergencies. These kits are easy to carry in a backpack, diaper bag, or purse and contain a shot of epinephrine that just might save your child's life if she accidentally eats something that causes her body to go into anaphylactic shock. Have one for home, school, and travel to ensure that medicine is always close by. A medical ID bracelet or necklace is also a good idea for the severely allergic child.

FOOD POISONING

No one likes to think about the foods we eat causing our family harm. However, the Centers for Disease Control and Prevention estimates that 76 million Americans will get food poisoning this year. That's quite a few upset stomachs!

Bacteria, like *Staph*, salmonella, or *E.coli*, cause the majority of cases. Because bacteria are invisible to the eye, the food looks and tastes normal. Fortunately, most cases of food poisoning are preventable. Ensuring good food hygiene and cooking habits can drastically decrease the incidence of this problem. Cooking meats at the proper temperature; avoiding raw, unwashed fruits and vegetables; and ensuring eggs have a firm yolk and white are all ways to keep the family safe from food-poisoning bacteria.

There are some food-borne toxins, like botulism, that are extremely dangerous if picked up in foods. Of the 120 botulism cases reported each year, nearly three-fourths are infants who get it from improperly prepared honey.

Symptoms of food poisoning are stomach cramps, diarrhea, and vomiting, usually within one to six hours after eating the offending foods. These symptoms generally last 12 to 24 hours.

NATURAL CHOICES
Keeping food safe is the best way to prevent an unpleasant occurrence of food poisoning. Here are some tips for family outings where food is packed:

■ Cool food is safer food. Pack extra ice packs when transporting perishables and avoid flimsy Styrofoam coolers.

■ Separate raw and cooked food. Seal meat tightly to prevent juices from contaminating other foods.

■ Time it, and then toss it. If spoilable food has been packed for over four hours and not eaten, it's better to get rid of it than risk food poisoning the family.

■ Use plastic wrap for better insulation. Studies show that double-wrapped foods stay fresher and cooler than those wrapped in aluminum foil.

OVER-THE-COUNTER PRODUCTS
When your child is throwing up and has diarrhea, the bells should go off that now is the time to be certain he drinks lots of liquids. The child's small body can't afford to lose these important fluids and still function normally. Stop all foods except clear liquids. High-calorie, high-electrolyte drinks like Pedialyte should be encouraged in small sips. If Pedialyte isn't available, try water, flat soda, or ginger ale.

For children over the age of six, the over-the-counter product Imodium-AD (loperamide) is often effective in just one dose for diarrhea and the stomach cramping that goes along with it.

DOCTOR VISITS
A visit to the doctor is in order if the child has a high fever, bloody diarrhea, or diarrhea lasting longer than two to three days for a young

child and 12 to 24 hours for a young infant. It is also in order if your child seems extremely weak and lethargic.

Prescription antinausea medicines, like Phenergan (promethazine), are often prescribed in suppository form for those who can't keep anything down.

One immediate concern is dehydration (see Dehydration, pg. 195). Check the skin for a "bread-dough" feeling—where an area of the child's skin remains indented if touched or pinched. Also check for any unusual dryness. Infants may have a sunken spot on the top of their head if they are losing too much water. At the hospital, the child may be given intravenous fluids to replace what has been lost.

GAS

Infant gas, or flatulence, is usually caused by a baby's new digestive system learning to cope with the process of turning milk products into fuel for the body. Breast milk and infant formula both contain proteins and milk sugars that must be broken down in the stomach. Gas is very common in babies. It affects almost half of all newborns within the first two months of life and generally goes away on its own, or becomes less frequent and painful, as little systems mature.

An excess of baby gas may be a signal that a baby is lactose intolerant (see Lactose Intolerance, pg. 262) or that the baby may have a sensitivity to certain ingredients in milk. Baby gas can also be brought on when a little screamer swallows big gulps of air with every yell. This excessive gulping of air builds up pressure in the child's stomach, making the little one feel extremely uncomfortable.

And what goes in must come out. While crying is one symptom of excess gas, an infant may also show discomfort by pulling her legs up tight against the body or lying in a curled position. Normally, the ritual of frequent burping will help expel the gas. However, there may be times when the baby just can't get rid of the gas and needs help from you.

NATURAL CHOICES

Many cases of mild baby gas can be resolved by simply moving the little one around until the gas is expelled. Here is one method for non-drug home treatment you might try: Lay your baby on her back on your lap with her head resting on your knees and her legs toward you. Gently pump her legs up and down in a bicycling motion. This helps move the gas out of the tummy where it is causing discomfort.

You should also burp your baby every three to five minutes during bottle feedings, or between breastfeedings, to prevent gas buildup and pain. Bottlefeeding can cause more bubbles in your baby's tummy than breastfeeding because your baby gets more air while drinking. On the other hand, babies can become gassy when breastfeeding because of the foods that are eaten by Mom. Broccoli and cabbage are just two of the foods that can cause baby gas in your infant. When it's the baby's food source that is to blame for all the gas, it may be necessary to switch formulas to find the right match for her system.

OVER-THE-COUNTER PRODUCTS

If your baby begins showing symptoms when you suspect gas, such as crying constantly or lying in a fetal position, give the doctor a call before you try the over-the-counter gas remedies. There may be a more serious medical problem brewing. The problem will likely be resolved by a trip to the drug store's "baby gas" department, but with little ones, it's best to be certain of the cause before giving them any medication.

Products like Infant's Mylicon Drops will give rapid relief to the discomfort and fussiness associated with the buildup of gas bubbles in the baby's stomach. The active ingredient simethecone works gently to break down gas bubbles in minutes. These drops are considered safe for infants because the medicine is not absorbed into your baby's system. The dosing of Infant's Mylicon Drops for babies under two years is 0.3ml four times daily after meals and at bedtime, or as directed by a physician. There is even a nonstaining formula with no artificial colors. The dosage can also be mixed with one ounce of cool water, infant formula, or other suitable liquids to make it more palatable for a baby.

DOCTOR VISITS

If your infant shows signs of discomfort after over-the-counter products have been tried, consult the doctor. Your pediatrician will have the right answers if the over-the-counter products just aren't quite enough to stop the painful gas. Some infants may require more relief than the over-the-counter remedies can provide. Small doses of medicines like Reglan (metoclopromide) can slow down the motion of the stomach enough to give it time to properly digest the food.

GERMAN MEASLES

German measles, also called rubella or three-day measles, is a viral illness with symptoms of a mild fever, swollen glands at the back of the head and behind the ears, and a skin rash. It is seen rarely today in the United States due to the MMR vaccine.

German measles may begin with one or two days of mild fever (99° F to 100° F) and swollen glands. On the second or third day, a rash appears that begins at the hairline and spreads downward on the rest of the body. As the rash spreads downward on the body, it usually clears on the face.

The German measles rash appears as either pink or light red spots, which may merge to form evenly colored patches. The rash doesn't itch, and lasts up to five days, with the average duration being three days. As the rash passes, the affected skin may be shed in flakes.

Someone infected with German measles is most contagious starting a few days before the rash develops until five to seven days after it first appears. A child usually develops symptoms 14 to 21 days after exposure to the virus. However, as many as 25 to 50 percent of those infected with the German measles virus do not develop any symptoms. All children infected with German measles are contagious whether or not they have symptoms. Any pregnant woman who has been exposed to German measles should contact her obstetrician immediately.

NATURAL CHOICES

Children, teens, and adults with German measles should not attend day care, school, or work or be around other people, especially pregnant women, for at least seven days after the rash first appears.

While the virus runs its course, the key is keeping your little one as comfortable as possible, using the following tips:

■ Stock the refrigerator with liquids your child enjoys. Water is best, but fruit juices and high-electrolyte energy drinks, like Power-Ade, Pedialyte, or Infalyte, will also help replenish fluids lost from the fever.

■ Place cool compresses on your child's forehead, back, and chest to help ease the feverish discomfort.

OVER-THE-COUNTER PRODUCTS

You probably already have on hand many of the over-the-counter medicines that can help your child feel more comfortable. Pain relievers/fever reducers, like Children's Tylenol (acetaminophen) or Children's Motrin (ibuprofen), are good choices for body aches and fevers.

DOCTOR VISITS

The MMR vaccine protects against infection with the measles, mumps, and rubella viruses. Your child should receive two doses of the MMR vaccine, first at his first birthday and a booster dose when he is four years old. Children who have had a life-threatening allergic reaction to gelatin, to the antibiotic neomycin, or to a previous dose of MMR vaccine should not receive this vaccine.

Mild side effects that your child may have seven to 12 days after receiving the MMR vaccine include fever, mild rash, and swelling of the glands in the cheeks or neck. Also be on the lookout for more serious side effects, including febrile seizures, temporary pain and stiffness in the joints, or a temporary low platelet count.

GINGIVITIS

This condition most often affects teens and older children with permanent teeth, but good dental habits from an early age can prevent this condition from ever occurring. Gingivitis is an inflammation of the gums, also called gingiva. The gums look red and swollen, and can bleed very easily. If untreated, gingivitis can cause long-term mouth damage when this inflammation spreads to the tooth and possibly deeper into the bone. Your child's teeth can be loosened and even lost if this condition does not receive proper medical attention.

The cause of gingivitis is improper brushing and flossing to remove plaque, the sticky, bacteria-filled film that covers the tooth enamel. If plaque is not removed within 72 hours, it hardens into tartar and becomes very difficult to remove. Getting rid of this plaque is key to preventing gingivitis.

Going through the hormonal changes of puberty and taking some medications, like Dilantin (phenytoin) or birth control pills, can make gingivitis worse. Once this condition is diagnosed, it may take several weeks of treatment before it is eliminated completely. Frequent checkups by the dentist are a must.

NATURAL CHOICES
Gingivitis is easily preventable and steps should be taken before home treatment is necessary. Proper brushing and flossing techniques keep plaque to a minimum. Have your child brush and floss twice daily and after meals when possible. Also have your child get a professional cleaning at least twice a year.

Gingivitis can be reversed in nearly all cases when proper plaque control is practiced.

In some rare cases, a vitamin deficiency is found to be the cause of gingivitis. If this is the case, add extra vitamin C to the diet, such as by drinking orange juice, which may be enough. Folic acid has also been shown to have beneficial effects for some individuals. Find a good multivitamin for your child and encourage him to take it every day. Vitaball is a new gum-ball vitamin that children really seem to favor.

OVER-THE-COUNTER PRODUCTS

For children over the age of six with gingivitis, the use of toothpastes that combine tartar-control pyrophosphates and the antibacterial triclosan, like Colgate Total, has shown great effects in limiting the amount of new tartar formed on teeth.

Look for toothpastes that carry the American Dental Association's Seal of Acceptance. This indicates that the toothpaste has met ADA criteria for safety and effectiveness. Be sure to read the manufacturer's label carefully. The ingredients in some toothpastes are not recommended for children under a certain age.

DOCTOR VISITS

For advanced cases of gingivitis, your child's dentist may prescribe a dental rinse called Peridex (chlorhexidine). This rinse works to decrease bacteria in the mouth and control plaque accumulation on the teeth. Be sure to follow the package directions carefully as this medication may stain the teeth if not used correctly.

Antibiotics, including doxycycline, tetracycline, and minocycline, may also be used to treat gum disease, as determined by your child's dentist. These work to reduce or temporarily eliminate the bacteria associated with gingivitis.

HAY FEVER

Hay fever, also called allergic rhinitis or seasonal allergies, describes all types of allergies caused by pollens, grasses, cottonwoods, and ragweed. Hay fever symptoms also include itchy, runny noses and scratchy, watery eyes.

The prevalence of hay fever may depend on your geographical area or environmental conditions. When the trees and grasses in your area produce pollen for longer periods, such as in warmer climates, there is a longer season for hay fever.

Hay fever doesn't have to be limited to outside conditions, either. It can also refer to an allergy to common household allergens, like pet hair and dander, dust mites, mold, or feathers. Because these allergies tend to occur year round instead of just seasonally, these are more commonly referred to as perennial allergies.

Both seasonal and perennial hay fevers will make themselves known to your child with symptoms of sneezing, a runny nose, swollen sinuses, itchy, watery eyes, and sometimes a headache from the sinus pressure.

NATURAL CHOICES

Completely avoiding the cause of a hay fever allergy is often impossible. A few tips for minimizing exposure to those pesky pollens and other allergens that contribute to your child's misery include:

- Knowing the pollen counts before your child steps outdoors and having your child stay inside on bad days, if possible.

- Using the air conditioner whenever possible, especially when a hay fever attack is in full swing.

- Having your child avoid smoky, stuffy places, which can irritate hay fever and maybe even cause a hay fever episode.

- Letting someone else comb the dog and cat, and then having your child stay away for a while after they're done, so the dander will have a chance to settle somewhere other than his nose.

■ Making your home dust-mite unfriendly by removing old and musty carpets and vacuuming often.

■ Not using feather pillows, but opting instead for man-made "hypoallergenic" products.

OVER-THE-COUNTER PRODUCTS

Headaches and body aches from the sinus pressure often associated with hay fever can be treated at home with children's Tylenol (acetaminophen) or Motrin (ibuprofen).

For hay fever prevention in children over six years, you might try cromolyn sodium. Found over-the-counter in products like Nasalcrom, this medication stops an allergy before it begins. However, it won't be effective once the allergic reaction has begun and it takes several days to a week of constant use before the full allergy prevention effect is in place. The active ingredient cromolyn is safe to use with other allergy medicines as well.

Antihistamines, like Benadryl (diphenhydramine), are available in both liquid and chewable forms. This medicine has been the allergy staple for years. Many doctors still recommend this as the top over-the-counter product for controlling allergy symptoms. However, newer nonsedating antihistamines, like Claritin (loratidine), are now available without a prescription for use in children. The liquid and quick-dissolving Reditabs work well for children over six years old.

DOCTOR VISITS

First, your child's allergist needs to know which allergens are causing the problems. It is impossible to keep the little one away from all pollens, so an allergy skin test may be required to pinpoint the problem.

Your child's doctor may take a blood test to see if there are antibodies present. Antibodies are produced in the body whenever we are exposed to an allergen. The test will help to determine exactly what is causing the allergic reaction. The doctor will check a specific allergen against the number and type of antibodies present (such as IgE antibodies) and decide if this allergen is the culprit. Once your child's doctor knows what is causing the problem, you must help your child learn to stay away from it. Avoidance of the allergen(s) causing the problem is the most effective treatment of hay fever.

Seasonal hay fever may require prescription medicines for the older child. Nasal steroids, like Nasacort (triamcinolone) or Beconase AQ (beclomethasone), help to decrease the swelling of nasal membranes and make breathing easier for your child.

HEAD LICE

The phrase "Your child has head lice" may just be one of the most upsetting things a parent can read on papers sent home from school. It is important to realize that head lice don't visit because your child is dirty, unwashed, or not cared for properly. Head lice are the second most communicable condition among children after the common cold. More than 10 million cases of head lice infestation are reported each year.

Head lice appear on the hair shafts and in the scalp as tiny, white, grayish-white, or yellowish insects. The female louse (singular for lice) lays five or ten eggs every day at the base of hair shafts at the scalp. The eggs are called nits and are strongly attached to the hair shaft. Head lice are most often found behind the ears and at the back of the neck. The lice feed on blood every three to six hours. This feeding can cause itching and the child's scalp may appear red, but in most cases there are no symptoms.

NATURAL CHOICES

The most common ways head lice are spread are through the sharing of hats, combs or, scarves, and through close contact among little heads. If your child has been exposed to lice, wash all bedding, hats, and scarves in hot water. Combs and brushes may be placed in a mild solution of water and bleach to ensure the nits are completely cleared. Check the hair of other family members frequently to ensure the lice haven't spread.

It's not clear whether herbal treatments, such as tea tree oil, lavender, or rosemary oil, really kill lice. It may be best not to try them until studies have shown whether they work—and whether they're safe. Current research suggests that combing your hair frequently in an attempt to remove lice and their eggs is also not an effective form of treatment.

OVER-THE-COUNTER PRODUCTS

Public consumer groups and the journal *Pediatrics* advise use of the over-the-counter permethrin product called Nix. This is a cream rinse made by the folks at Warner Lambert. Its active ingredient dissolves the sticky coating holding the nit in place on the hair shaft. Nix kills lice in ten to 15 minutes with a success rate of 97 to 99 percent in 14 days. Applied to towel-dried hair after shampooing, it is left in place for ten to 15 minutes, and then immediately rinsed out.

Rid and A-200 use the active ingredient pyrethrin to kill lice. Pyrethrin is a chemical extracted from the chrysanthemum flower that acts like an insecticide, destroying the nervous system of lice, and killing them within ten to 20 minutes, along with 75 percent of their nits. Redness and itching are common side effects of pyrethrin, especially for children with a ragweed allergy.

After using an over-the-counter product to treat lice, scalp itching is common. You may want to use corticosteroid creams, like hydrocortisone, or calamine lotion to relieve the itching. For severe itching, oral antihistamines, such as Benadryl (diphenhydramine), may be used.

DOCTOR VISITS

Prescription shampoos, like Quell (lindane), also known as gamma benzene hexachloride, may be prescribed in severe cases of infestation. It is toxic to the child's nervous system if used incorrectly and has been reported to cause severe seizures in children. Aplastic anemia, leukemia, and other blood diseases have also been associated with lindane. Consumer groups have called for a ban on the drug. The U.S. Food and Drug Administration permits the sale of lindane, but has ordered that its most severe warning—the "black box" label—be put on the drug's box.

A prescription medication is also available called Stromectol (ivermectin). This drug is commonly used to treat worm infections, but studies show promise for lice as well. It is an oral tablet and in some cases can be used when topical treatment using two or more approved shampoos or lotions has failed to get rid of lice. However, it has not been studied in children weighing less than 35 pounds.

HEAT STROKE/HEAT EXHAUSTION

Heat stroke occurs when the body is unable to regulate its temperature. The body's temperature rises rapidly, the sweating mechanism fails, and the body is unable to cool down. Body temperature may rise to 106° F or higher within ten to 15 minutes. Heat stroke can cause death or permanent disability if emergency treatment is not provided. Warning signs of heat stroke vary but may include the following:

- An extremely high body temperature (above 103° F, orally)

- Red, hot, and dry skin, with no sweating

- A rapid, strong pulse

- A throbbing headache

- Dizziness

- Nausea

- Confusion

- Unconsciousness

If your child exhibits any of these signs, you may be dealing with a life-threatening emergency. Sometimes a heat stroke victim's muscles will begin to twitch uncontrollably. If this happens, keep the child from injuring himself, but do not place any object in the mouth and do not give fluids. If there is vomiting, make sure the airway remains open by turning the child on his or her side. Have someone call for immediate medical assistance while you begin cooling the child. Do the following:

- Get the child to a shady area.

- Cool the child rapidly using whatever methods you can. For example, immerse him in a tub of cool water, place him in a cool shower, spray him with cool water from a garden hose, or sponge him down with cool water. If the humidity is low, wrap him in a cool, wet sheet and fan vigorously.

■ Monitor body temperature, and continue cooling efforts until the oral body temperature drops to 101°F or 102°F.

■ If emergency medical personnel are delayed, call the hospital emergency room for further instructions.

Heat exhaustion is a milder form of heat-related illness that can develop after several days of exposure to high temperatures and inadequate or unbalanced replacement of fluids. Young children and the elderly are especially susceptible to this illness. The warning signs of heat exhaustion include the following:

■ Heavy sweating

■ Paleness

■ Muscle cramps

■ Tiredness

■ Weakness

■ Dizziness

■ Headache

■ Nausea or vomiting

■ Fainting

The skin may be cool and moist. The pulse rate will be fast and weak, and breathing will be fast and shallow. If heat exhaustion is untreated, it may progress to heat stroke. Bring your child to the doctor right away if symptoms worsen or last longer than one hour.

NATURAL CHOICES

Keeping the child's body cool is the best way to prevent heat-related illness. Here are steps to take for home prevention:

■ Keep air-conditioning on when the temperature is in the high nineties. Electric fans provide some comfort, but will not prevent heat-related illness. Air-conditioning is the strongest protective factor against heat-related illness. Exposure to air-conditioning for even a few hours a day will reduce the risk for heat-related illness.

■ Put the child in a cool shower or bath.

■ During hot weather, your child will need to drink more liquid than his thirst indicates. Provide large quantities of water and ensure it is consumed.

■ Consider visiting a shopping mall, public library, or other air-conditioned space for a few hours.

■ Choose lightweight, light-colored, loose-fitting clothing for the child.

OVER-THE-COUNTER PRODUCTS

Electrolyte replacement liquids, a combination of water, sodium, potassium, chloride, and sugars that help the body recover from fluid loss by replacing what was lost, come in a variety of favorite flavors. Putting a bottle of this liquid in the refrigerator or freezer to keep it cold increases the palatability and will help cool hot bodies. Brands available from the pharmacy shelf include Pedialyte and Infalyte. Keep in mind that once opened, a bottle is only good for 48 hours before it should be discarded.

As an extra special treat on hot days, try Pedialyte Freezer Pops. They contain the right mix of eloctrolytes to replace those lost from excessive sweating and heat acclimation.

DOCTOR VISITS

Prompt medical attention is of primary importance when a heat-related illness is suspected. Medical personnel will work to cool the body and bring the body temperature back to normal. If hospitalization is required, intravenous fluids and salts are administered to bring body fluids back into balance.

HIVES

If your child comes in contact with something that she is allergic to, it triggers a condition called hives. Environmental factors like illness and emotional stress can also result in hives. Hives occur in part because the body's immune system is set up with an extensive force of guards called mast cells that prevent attack by foreign substances. When the body is exposed to something it detects as harmful, the mast cells become kamikazes and explode. This tiny explosion releases a chemical called histamine into the body and an allergic reaction follows. Hives appear as raised, red, and itchy areas of the skin referred to as wheals.

Hives aren't contagious and are pretty easy to figure out. If your daughter has just eaten something unusual, has been in the sun, or has just been rolling in the grass, and she breaks out with red, itchy areas of skin, she probably has hives. Most cases of hives can be traced to one, or more than one, of the below:

- **Nuts:** peanuts, walnuts, or Brazil nuts

- **Seafood:** shrimp, clams, or other shellfish

- **Medications:** penicillin, flu vaccines, or tetanus shots

- **Foods:** strawberries, milk, or wheat

- **Insect bites/stings:** bees, ants, wasps, or hornets

- **Environmental factors:** cold, heat, sunshine, or latex

- **Emotional/physical stress:** infections, exercise, or home or school stress

It is common for hives to appear and then disappear within the same day, especially if what causes the allergy is only in contact with the child for a short time. However, if the agent causing the reaction isn't removed, hives can last for several weeks. It is important to be cautious when your child experiences a case of hives for the first time. Hives can be one of the first symptoms of anaphylactic shock (see Anaphylactic Shock, pg. 138). If the hives progress into swelling of the throat or tongue causing difficulty breathing, call 911 right away.

NATURAL CHOICES
The first course of action with hives is to determine what is causing the reaction and keep your child away from it. Histamine, the body's itch chemical, is released more readily when the area with hives is warmed or rubbed, so avoid exposing the itchy area to heat or rubbing it. Also try the following:

- To cool and soothe itchy areas, use cold rag compresses or resealable plastic bags filled with ice water.

- Add a cup of plain oatmeal to a lukewarm bath for bathtime relief from the itch of hives.

■ Keep your child's fingernails clipped short to prevent scratching and possible skin infections.

OVER-THE-COUNTER PRODUCTS

Benadryl (diphenhydramine) products are used for itchy rashes. You'll find Benadryl in liquid form for younger children; in chewable tablets for older kids; and in itch-relieving sprays, creams, and gel forms for children over the age of 12.

Calamine lotion and hydrocortisone creams are also very effective for controlling the itch.

Aveeno oatmeal bath is another good product to have around the house. The soothing action of the oatmeal acts to cool the skin and ease the itch. Because the oatmeal products can make the bathtub slippery, it is a very good idea to put down a tub mat to prevent a nasty fall.

DOCTOR VISITS

Hives may be just an unpleasant temporary annoyance, or may be a sign that something more serious is occuring. If it is your child's first case of hives or an unusually severe or long-lasting episode, it is a good idea to visit a doctor as soon as possible. Some cases of hives require corticosteroids, like prednisolone, or prescription antihistamines, like hydroxyzine.

If your child has a case of hives that doesn't respond to antihistamines or corticosteroids, or if there is accompanying swelling of the airways hindering your child's ability to breathe, she may need to be treated quickly with an epinephrine (adrenaline) shot. This drug will quickly open the breathing passages and could save your child's life. Children with a past reaction that included hives should always carry an anaphylaxis kit, like Epi-Pen, to prevent a more serious reaction from occurring.

IMPETIGO

Impetigo is a highly contagious skin infection caused by either *Staph* or *Strep* bacteria and spread by person to person contact. It is commonly seen on the faces of young children, especially around the areas of the nose and mouth.

The infection begins as small, fluid-filled blisters in an area where the skin has been damaged by scratching or scraped. The fluid in the blisters contains bacteria, so once the blisters break, the infection spreads rapidly. The itchy sores quickly increase in size and can cover a large area of the face with a golden scabby layer.

Impetigo runs its course in seven to ten days and usually causes no further problems. However, if certain forms of *Strep* bacteria are the cause, a more serious kidney condition called glomerulonephritis can develop.

NATURAL CHOICES

Because of the highly contagious nature of this skin infection, it is vitally important to limit contact of other family members to the infected child's towels, bedclothes, or personal clothing. Favorite toys and areas where the child spends time should be disinfected frequently. If only one family member has impetigo, everyone in the household should follow the same sanitary routine.

For mild cases of impetigo, simply washing the infected area carefully with a gentle antibacterial soap and warm water can help soften the crusty areas and limit the spread of bacteria.

Trimming fingernails short can help control the spread to other parts of the body from bacteria under the nails, as well as preventing new skin trauma in which the bacteria can find a home.

OVER-THE-COUNTER PRODUCTS

If the infection is relatively minor, the doctor may recommend an over-the-counter cream or ointment containing antibiotics specific for the skin. However, some studies have shown that these are not powerful enough to kill the bacteria completely. If your doctor gives the okay for an over-the-counter product, the mild antibiotic cream bacitracin is a good choice. After spreading on the antibiotic, covering the affected area with a Band-Aid or gauze can serve to protect the sores and prevent the spread of the bacteria.

Each day care facility or school has their own rules, but typically an infected child should be kept away from others until he has been treated with antibiotic creams for 48 hours or has been taking oral antibiotics for 24 hours. In mild cases of impetigo, the child can attend school if the sores are covered with a Band-Aid and an antibiotic cream or ointment. Please make day care or school workers aware that your child has this infection to prevent a major outbreak among all the children there.

DOCTOR VISITS

A serious complication of impetigo is glomerulonephritis, a dangerous kidney disease. When occurring at the same time as impetigo, symptoms of this condition requiring prompt medical treatment, include stomach upset, headaches, a puffy face, or lower than normal urinary output. The doctor will take a sample of the bacteria from your child, and if it is *Strep*, she will be on the lookout for glomerulonephritis.

The prescription medication most often prescribed for impetigo is the antibacterial cream Bactroban (mupirocin). For more involved cases, an oral antibiotic like amoxicillin or erythromycin may be needed to control the spread of the infection. Both the cream and antibiotic may be needed in severe cases.

JAUNDICE

Nearly 60 percent of full-term newborns develop jaundice on the second or third day after birth. That's quite a few infants turning yellow! Jaundice, also called hyperbilirubinemia, is an unusually high blood level of the yellow pigment bilirubin. Bilirubin is formed from broken down hemoglobin proteins in the blood. Typically newborns have a larger amount of hemoglobin than adults or older children. Normally, bilirubin circulates to the liver and is excreted as a part of normal bile. However, the baby's immature intestinal system sometimes can't get rid of this pigment and their skin appears yellow. The skin and whites of the eyes have a yellowish tinge, but it helps to view the baby in normal, not artificial, light to determine if this is a true color change. This type of jaundice, often called normal jaundice, is almost always harmless and usually disappears after the first week.

However, there are other forms of jaundice, which if not treated quickly, can be dangerous for infants and young children. Blood poisoning and erythroblastosis fetalis, in which there is an incompatibility of the child's blood and the mother's, can appear as newborn jaundice, but must be treated immediately.

NATURAL CHOICES

Breastfeeding is often responsible for bringing on or even prolonging newborn jaundice. This is called breast milk jaundice and is thought to occur due to a specific substance in breast milk limiting the baby's ability to excrete bilirubin. For treatment of this type of jaundice, take your baby off the breast milk and switch him to formula for one to two days while continuing to pump milk. This will decrease the signs of jaundice and give the baby's body time to begin producing bacteria to begin breaking down bilirubin naturally.

Mild, uncomplicated jaundice is usually left to run its course on its own. The baby's body begins to produce the important bilirubin-digesting bacteria and the problem soon solves itself. Frequent feedings, especially when breastfeeding, ensure food is passing through the baby's system quickly before the enzymes limiting the breakdown of bilirubin have an opportunity to be absorbed into the blood.

If the doctor feels the child's bilirubin level isn't high enough for admittance to the hospital, he may recommend putting the baby near a window for as much filtered sunshine as possible. This home phototherapy changes bilirubin into substances the infant's body can process and thereby decreases the symptoms of jaundice.

OVER-THE-COUNTER PRODUCTS
If you suspect jaundice, don't try to treat it at home. Because there is the possibility of more serious causes of jaundice, over-the-counter products are not recommended.

DOCTOR VISITS
Babies whose skin appears yellow should be brought in for a doctor's visit to rule out causes that are more serious. High blood bilirubin levels are treated with phototherapy under bilirubin lights, also called bililights. These blue lights change bilirubin into compounds much easier for the infant's body to process naturally. For infants with severe jaundice, blood transfusions may be required to exchange fresh blood with that saturated with bilirubin.

JOCK ITCH

Jock itch, also called tinea cruris, is a fungal infection of the ringworm variety in the groin area. Both boys and girls can get it, but it is more commonly seen in your young male athlete. He'll pick this up from the irritation of the moist groin area and the growth of the *Trichophyton rubrum* fungus. Jock straps and tight uniforms contribute to the problem.

Jock itch appears with a rash of small, red, ring-like bumps. The bumps can produce small liquid-filled blisters that are very itchy. They cover the groin area and the external genitalia. They may also spread to the inner thighs and folds of the skin. For most cases of jock itch, home treatment will take care of the problem within a week.

NATURAL CHOICES

Jock itch can be prevented by having your child keep his skin dry and clean. Showering often, especially after sweaty exercise, is important. He should also avoid wearing tight underwear. Frequently washing his exercise clothes and underwear can also reduce the chance for a fungal growth.

While waiting for over-the-counter antifungals to do the job, it is important that your child keep the groin area as dry as possible. If your child is wearing a jock strap and/or tight briefs, he should consider switching to boxers until the infection clears. This will give the groin area more opportunity to stay dry and the annoying itch time to go away.

OVER-THE-COUNTER PRODUCTS

For home treatment of jock itch, use a nonprescription antifungal cream or powder, like Micatin, Tinactin, Lamisil, or Lotrimin. These contain miconazole, terbinafine, or clotrimazole as their active ingredients. For cases of jock itch when the intense itchiness becomes a problem, applying a light coating of hydrocortisone cream or ointment to the rash should help quite a bit. This may be used in addition to an over-the-counter antifungal medicine.

There are many different products on the shelf, and it may be difficult to decide which form to use. Powders are good for places where sweating is a problem, like in the folds of skin or where underwear is in constant contact with the skin. Sprays are the easiest to apply, but may be cold and may waste medicine unless you have great aim. Creams or lotions can be applied directly to the rash and are generally thought to be the most effective. Wash the rash with soap and water, remove any pieces of dried skin, and spread an antifungal cream over the rash. Apply the cream beyond the edge or border of the rash.

Lamisil AT (terbinafine) in the spray pump is a convenient and effective way to treat jock itch for children 12 years and older. Wash the affected skin with soap and water and dry completely before applying. Spray the affected area once a day—morning or night—for one week or as directed by a doctor. Don't stop applying the medication just because the symptoms go away. If symptoms do not improve after two weeks, call the doctor.

DOCTOR VISITS

Prescription antifungals may be used for the case of jock itch that doesn't respond to over-the-counter products. Medications, like griseofulvin (Grifulvin-V), terbinafine (Lamisil), itraconazole (Sporanox), or ketoconazole (Nizoral), have all shown similar rates of success when taken as directed.

If there is the possibility of a secondary bacterial infection, the doctor may also prescribe an antibacterial cream or ointment for the skin, like Bactroban (mupirocin), until the infection clears.

KAWASAKI DISEASE

Kawasaki disease is an inflammatory condition of the blood vessels and heart that usually occurs in children younger than five years of age, and most commonly presents between the ages 18 months and two years. Approximately 3,000 cases occur each year in the United States. Children of Japanese and Korean background have a higher incidence, but it can occur in all ethnic and racial groups. The symptoms can be difficult to diagnose as the disease occurs in several stages:

■ The first symptom is a high fever, often higher than 104° F, which lasts for at least five days. The fever may last from ten to 25 days.

■ Within the first day or two, the child may develop the eye infection conjunctivitis with discharge.

■ In about 50 percent of cases, there will be swelling over the neck, representing an enlargement of the lymph nodes. Hands and feet may also swell.

■ In 80 percent of children, a rash is present over the chest and abdomen and at times over the arms and legs. It is usually red, but no blistering should be present. Peeling of the skin may be noted around the diaper area.

■ The lips become cracked, red, and dry. The tongue swells and resembles a strawberry.

■ In the second phase, peeling of the skin starting at the nail margins of the fingers and toes may be seen.

■ Some children experience joint pain, diarrhea, vomiting, and abdominal pain.

The importance of making a diagnosis between five to ten days from the onset of fever is to prevent later complications that may involve the arteries of the heart.

Heart disease is the most serious complication of Kawasaki disease and causes aneurysms or bulging in the small arteries around the heart, usually several weeks after the onset of fever. Untreated, it is one of the most common causes of heart attacks in children. Proper treatment reduces the risk of developing aneurysms to only two to four percent of children with Kawasaki disease.

Diagnosis of Kawasaki disease requires the presence of at least five of the symptoms discussed above, (fever, red eyes, red lips/throat, rash, swelling of hands/feet, lymph node enlargement in the neck), and blood tests that confirm the presence of an inflammation. However, in many instances, your child may not have all the symptoms required to make the diagnosis and may still have an atypical case of Kawasaki disease. It is important to try to diagnose the disease with some certainty within ten days and start treatment to decrease the incidence of complications involving the heart.

Most patients, if they do not develop the heart complications, recover completely without any long-term effects. Children with heart aneurysms may also recover fully, depending on their severity. Overall, about 50 percent of aneurysms resolve in one to two years.

NATURAL CHOICES

Because the cause for Kawasaki disease is not known, there is no prevention at this time. Home treatment is not recommended. Prompt medical attention at the hospital is called for.

OVER-THE-COUNTER PRODUCTS

This is one of the few conditions among children when the use of aspirin is recommended. During the convalescent phase of the disease, doctors often prescribe aspirin to decrease the inflammation in the body. It is important that you talk to your physician before stopping the aspirin, even if it has been several months and your child is doing well. You should also discuss with your physician what to do if your child develops a viral illness due to the risk of Reye's syndrome (see Reye's Syndrome, pg. 282). A child who has suffered Kawasaki disease also should receive the influenza vaccine each year.

DOCTOR VISITS

Blood tests done early in the course of the disease will usually show signs of inflammation, represented by an increased ESR (erythrocyte sedimentation rate) or CRP (C-reactive protein) and white blood cell count. An electrocardiogram is useful initially to rule out abnormalities of the heart. Other disorders that may be difficult to distinguish from Kawasaki include Steven Johnson syndrome, an allergic reaction, scarlet fever, and toxic shock syndrome.

Treatment is usually begun as soon as a diagnosis is made. Your child will likely be hospitalized and have an intravenous line placed. Intravenous immunoglobulin (IVIG) is the treatment of choice and has been shown to dramatically decrease the incidence of heart problems if given within ten days. In most cases, fever and other symptoms resolve within 24 hours after initiating IVIG.

Your child should be seen by a cardiologist who will evaluate the condition of the heart with an echocardiogram or ultrasound of the heart, and an electrocardiogram. These tests will be repeated for several weeks to months, depending on the severity of illness.

The next phase is the convalescent stage, in which symptoms have gone away. It continues until the ESR has returned to normal, which is usually about six to eight weeks after the illness began. In addition to IVIG, your child will probably also be started on aspirin. The initial doses will be high for the first few weeks, and then decreased to a lower level, until the end of the convalescent stage. In children with heart problems, especially those with aneurysms, the dose will be continued for several months to years to prevent formation of clots in the damaged blood vessels.

LACTOSE INTOLERANCE

There are three different types of lactose intolerance in children: primary, secondary, and congenital. The type will determine whether it is something your child will outgrow or something that will be around forever. All types of lactose intolerance arise from the inability of the body to break down the milk sugar lactose. This occurs because the body fails to produce the enzyme lactase. Lactase breaks down lactose into a more usable form.

When this undigested milk sugar, or lactose, finds its way through the digestive tract, intestinal bacteria take over the job. This bacterial breakdown of lactose results in hydrogen gas, (which in turn results in *very* smelly) diarrhea and stomach pain. Other common indicators of lactose intolerance include nausea, cramps, and bloating, all of which begin about 30 minutes to two hours after eating or drinking foods containing lactose.

Primary lactose intolerance is the condition that usually begins around the ages of three to 13 and will continue through life. It seems that in certain populations—particularly those of Mediterranean, African, Asian, and Native American backgrounds—75 to 100 percent of the people experience this type of lactose intolerance. The reason these groups of people seem to be prone to lactose intolerance as they grow older is because the lactase enzyme levels in the body gradually decrease with age. This is thought to occur because historically they were not drinking milk after infancy.

Secondary lactose intolerance occurs because the area in the lining of the intestinal wall where lactase is produced is temporarily damaged. Certain antibiotics, pain-relieving medicines, like nonsteroidal anti-inflammatory drugs, or even a severe bout of diarrhea can cause this. This problem usually takes care of itself as soon as the intestinal lining has time to heal and begin production of the lactase enzyme again.

In congenital lactose intolerance, the intestine simply does not make the enzyme lactase. This is a rare condition and is usually diagnosed within the first week after birth. These infants must be fed lactose-free formulas to accommodate their systems and will need to continue using lactose-free products throughout their lives.

NATURAL CHOICES

Lactose intolerance has no cure. Symptoms can be treated, but avoidance of lactose-containing products is the best defense. With primary and secondary lactose intolerance, the focus must be on either eliminating lactose-containing foods from the diet entirely or adding the enzyme lactase to the system. For infants with secondary lactose intolerance, changing the formula from lactose to a soy base may improve the symptoms dramatically.

Yogurt with active cultures may be a good source of calcium for many children with lactose intolerance, even though it is fairly high in lactose. Evidence shows that the bacterial cultures used in making yogurt produce some of the lactase enzyme required for proper digestion. Look for "live, active cultures" on the label.

OVER-THE-COUNTER PRODUCTS

If your child reacts to very small amounts of lactose or has trouble limiting his intake of foods that contain lactose, products like Lactaid may
help. This product contains the enzyme lactase and should be taken just
before dairy products are consumed. Several commercial preparations
of lactase are available, including a liquid form for direct addition to
milk and a capsule form that may be swallowed or broken open and
sprinkled over food. Caplets and chewable tablets are also offered and
should be taken with the lactose-containing food. Adding lactase to regular milk, for example, has been shown to significantly reduce symptoms of milk intolerance. All of these methods for introducing lactase
into the body, whether by directly adding it to foods or by taking it in
tablet form, have a considerable effect in reducing the pain, gas, diarrhea, and bloating of lactose intolerance. Pick the method most appropriate and easiest for your child.

DOCTOR VISITS

To determine if your child's symptoms are caused by lactose intolerance, your child's doctor can perform one of several tests to resolve if
a true lactose intolerance is present or if another cause is the problem.
For infants, a stool acidity test may be used to measure the amount of
acid in the stool. When lactose from milk products reaches the colon
undigested and bacteria take over, high amounts of lactic acid are
produced that show up in this test.

For older children, the hydrogen breath test records the amount
of gas produced when an individual drinks a high-lactose beverage.
High levels of hydrogen gas equate to improper lactose digestion.

Another common test is the lactose intolerance test. To prepare
for this test, your child isn't allowed to eat or drink anything before
the test. He will then drink a high-lactose beverage. Blood samples
are taken over a two-hour period to determine how well his body di-

gests the lactose. Low blood sugar levels mean that little lactose has been broken down and lactose intolerance is diagnosed.

LYME DISEASE

Lyme disease is a bacterial infection transmitted by the bite of a tick. Either the deer tick in the Midwestern and Northeastern United States or the Western black-legged tick on the Pacific Coast can spread this disease. Children aged five to nine are most at risk. However, any child playing in tall grass, shrubs, or wooded areas may be bitten and infected. May, June, and July are the months when Lyme disease is contracted most often.

The bacteria *Borrelia burgdorferi* causes the infection and is most often transmitted by the tiny (pinhead-sized) nymph stage of the tick. These are difficult to notice until a red, bull's-eye rash appears around the area of the bite. If an infected tick stays attached to the skin for 36 to 48 hours, the risk of contracting Lyme disease increases greatly. Early signs of the disease may include a skin rash, body aches and pains, mild fever, and flu-like symptoms. However, a telltale rash is not always present, thus making diagnosis difficult.

NATURAL CHOICES
To decrease your child's chances of coming into contact with a tick, be sure that when they are playing outdoors in wooded or grassy areas they wear long-sleeved shirts, hats, and pants tucked into socks. If the clothing is also lightly colored, you will be able to

spot a tick more easily. Perform a tick check on children before bath time to ensure no ticks are present. Household pets should be checked often, as they may bring ticks inside the house. Talk to the veterinarian about medications for the dog and cat to prevent tick infestation.

To remove a tick on your child:

■ Wear protective gloves to prevent blood from the tick getting on your hands.

■ Use fine-point tweezers to grasp the tick as close to the skin as possible.

■ Pull gently. Avoid squeezing the body of the tick.

■ Clean the site of the bite, your hands, and the tweezers with disinfectant.

You also may want to place the tick in a small container, like a pill container, and bring it to your doctor, pharmacist, or veterinarian for identification. Never use a burned match, petroleum jelly, or nail polish to try to remove ticks. Contrary to popular belief, these methods are ineffective and may cause parts of the tick to become lodged under the skin.

OVER-THE-COUNTER PRODUCTS
For children undergoing antibiotic treatment for Lyme disease, home care should be focused on making the child more comfortable. Over-the-counter children's pain relievers, like Tylenol (acetaminophen) or Motrin (ibuprofen) help relieve body aches and flu-like symptoms while the prescription antibiotic takes care of the infection.

DOCTOR VISITS

If your child is bitten by a tick in one of the high-risk geographical areas, the doctor may start a short course of antibiotics as a prophylaxis (or prevention) of Lyme disease. However, the American Academy of Pediatrics maintains, "We do not recommend prophylactic antibiotics. The risk after tick exposure is very low. . . . There can be more harm done with the overuse of antibiotics in the attempt to prevent Lyme disease." (See The Antibiotic Epidemic, pg. 23). If your child is diagnosed at the early stages of Lyme disease, antibiotics can typically kill the bacteria and no further complications develop. Because the symptoms of Lyme disease mimic so many other conditions, your child's doctor may do a blood test to determine if Lyme disease is indeed the problem.

MEASLES

Measles, also called rubeola or red measles, is a viral infection with symptoms that include a high fever, cough, runny nose, red eyes that are very sensitive to light, irritability, and a distinctive red rash that begins on the neck and travels down the body. Another distinctive feature of measles is Koplik's spots, which are small red spots with white centers that appear inside the mouth.

Measles are transmitted when an infected person coughs or sneezes. The virus is most often spread when people first become ill, before the rash develops, and before they know they have the disease. Measles can be spread from five days before the rash breaks out to four days after the rash disappears. Thankfully, due to the MMR vaccine, this is one condition that we seldom see anymore in the United States.

NATURAL CHOICES

Because measles are a contagious condition, it's important that a sick child doesn't expose others to the condition. This may mean a few days at home alone and away from playmates who haven't had measles or those individuals who haven't been immunized. Typically, your child should be kept away from others until the rash has been gone for four days and she is feeling normal again.

While the virus runs its course, the key is keeping your little one as comfortable as possible. Consider doing the following:

■ Stock the refrigerator with liquids your child enjoys. Water is best, but fruit juices and high-electrolyte energy drinks, like PowerAde, Gatorade, or Pedialyte, also help replenish fluids lost from the fever.

■ Place cool compresses on the forehead, back, and chest to help ease the feverish discomfort.

■ As measles and the accompanying fever can make your child temporarily sensitive to bright light, close the blinds and curtains to keep the room darker and avoid harsh lighting until your child feels better.

OVER-THE-COUNTER PRODUCTS

You probably already have on hand many of the over-the-counter medicines that can help your child feel more comfortable. Pain relievers/fever reducers, like Children's Tylenol (acetaminophen) or Children's Motrin (ibuprofen), are good choices for body aches and fevers.

DOCTOR VISITS

The MMR vaccine, a combination of the measles, mumps and rubella viruses, protects against infection. Your child should receive two doses of the MMR vaccine, the first dose at his first birthday and a booster dose when he is four years old. Children who have had a life-threatening allergic reaction to gelatin, to the antibiotic neomycin, or to a previous dose of MMR vaccine should not receive this vaccine.

Mild side effects that your child may have seven to 12 days after receiving the MMR vaccine include, fever, mild rash, and swelling of the glands in the cheeks or neck. Also be on the lookout for more serious side effects, including febrile seizures (see Febrile Seizures, pg. 219), or pain and stiffness in the joints.

MUMPS

Mumps is a contagious viral condition seen rarely today in the United States due to the MMR vaccine. The mumps virus is spread when an infected person coughs and sneezes, as well as through contact with contaminated items, such as tissues, drinking glasses, and dirty hands. The virus is most often spread within a day or two before the first symptoms appear, although it can be spread any time from seven days before symptoms appear to nine days after symptoms appear.

The most common symptoms of mumps are a low-grade fever, abdominal pain, headache, and facial swelling. This facial swelling is caused by the swelling of the salivary glands. As a result, chewing and swallowing can become very painful. Complication of mumps can also include painful and swollen testicles in older boys, meningitis, and, uncommonly, inflammation of the brain, also called encephalitis. There is no cure or treatment for mumps. Home care focuses on making the child more comfortable.

NATURAL CHOICES

Children with mumps should not go to school, day care, or public places until nine days after the salivary glands first start to swell or three days after the swelling has gone down. It is not generally necessary to separate a child from the family, because by the time mumps is diagnosed, most household members have already been exposed.

If you or your child has mumps, call your local health department. The health department needs to record all cases of the illness. If you visit your doctor, he or she will report it for you.

While the virus runs its course, the key is keeping your little one as comfortable as possible by doing the following:

■ Stock the refrigerator with liquids your child enjoys. Water is best, but cool fruit juices and high-electrolyte energy drinks, like PowerAde or Gatorade for older children, or Pedialyte or Infalyte for the younger set, will also help replenish fluids lost from the fever.

■ Offer your child popsicles and easy-to-swallow cold liquids, like ice cream or gelatin, as eating may be unbearable.

■ Don't give sour foods or sour liquids, because the infected salivary glands are extremely sensitive to sour tastes.

■ Make an ice pack of cold water and ice in a resealable plastic bag and place it on the neck and throat.

OVER-THE-COUNTER PRODUCTS

You probably already have on hand many of the over-the-counter medicines that can help your child feel more comfortable. Pain relievers/fever reducers, like Children's Tylenol (acetaminophen) or Children's Motrin (ibuprofen), are good choices for body aches, swollen testicles, and fevers.

DOCTOR VISITS

The MMR vaccine protects against infection with the measles, mumps, and rubella viruses. Your child should receive two doses of the MMR vaccine, at his first birthday and a booster dose when he is four years old. Children who have had a life-threatening allergic reaction to gelatin, to the antibiotic neomycin, or to a previous dose of MMR vaccine should not receive this vaccine.

Mild side effects that your child may have seven to 12 days after receiving the MMR vaccine include fever, mild rash, or a swelling of the glands in the cheeks or neck. Also be on the lookout for more serious side effects, including febrile seizures (see Febrile Seizures, pg. 219), pain and stiffness in the joints, or a temporary low platelet count.

NAUSEA AND VOMITING

Technically, nausea is an unpleasant wave-like feeling in the back of the throat and/or stomach that may or may not result in vomiting. Vomiting occurs when stomach contents are forcefully emptied. Nausea and vomiting go hand in hand, but it is possible to feel nauseous without actually vomiting. An area of the brain called the vomiting center triggers both activities.

Both the feeling of nausea and the actual vomiting can be caused by an infection, like stomach flu; movement, like car sickness; pain; or irritation of the senses by certain smells and foods. During the act of vomiting or throwing up, your child's windpipe closes to prevent what's coming up from getting into the lungs, while his abdomen and diaphragm contract forcefully to push everything out quickly.

NATURAL CHOICES

Home treatment of nausea and vomiting should begin early. While nausea and vomiting usually stop when the cause of the problem is removed, it can become very serious when the child cannot keep any fluids down and becomes dehydrated (see Dehydration, pg. 195). It is important to ensure that fluids are replaced in your child's body as quickly as possible to avoid serious dehydration. Try to give small amounts of flat soda or clear, nondiet drinks like Sprite or 7-Up. Sugared drinks are better than plain water. Avoid high-acid drinks, like orange or grapefruit juice, that can cause more stomach discomfort.

OVER-THE-COUNTER PRODUCTS

Nausea, upset stomach, and vomiting all seem to occur precisely at the moment when all pharmacies in the vicinity close for the night. Having medicine around the house for such emergencies is always a good idea. A must for family first-aid kits is the liquid Emetrol. It works quickly for the relief of nausea and vomiting due to upset stomach from intestinal flu and stomach flu. This is safe for children over the age of two years because the active ingredient is not a drug, but a sugar solution of dextrose, levulose (fructose), and phosphoric acid. It soothes the tummy by decreasing the pressure within the stomach. The sugars work to delay the vomiting reflex. It tastes pretty good, too. However, because of the high sugar content, children with diabetes should avoid Emetrol.

Another popular choice is Pepto-Bismol. Pepto-Bismol is a bismuth salt that acts by coating the inside of the stomach to relieve the feeling of nausea. Children and teenagers who have or are recovering from chicken pox or flu should not use this medicine to treat nausea or vomiting due to the possibility of Reye's syndrome (see Reye's Syndrome, pg. 282).

Most over-the-counter antinausea medications for children over the age of 12 are designed to treat motion sickness and focus on the middle ear to restore balance. Look for names like Bonine (meclizine) or Dramamine (dimenhydrinate). The most common side effects are drowsiness and grogginess. Blurred vision and dry mouth are infrequent side effects, but may also occur.

If your child's nausea and vomiting episodes are unexplained or severe, or last longer than 12 hours, talk to the doctor before using over-the-counter antinausea products.

DOCTOR VISITS

If the nausea doesn't seem responsive to over-the-counter products or lasts more than 12 hours, it's time to call the doctor. Infants who are vomiting repeatedly should be seen by a physician right away. Do not give infants more than one or two ounces of plain water, as this may lead to electrolyte imbalances (see Electrolyte Imbalance, pg. 216). Instead, maintain hydration by using half-strength formula or an oral rehydration solution such as Pedialyte, given in frequent, small amounts. Start with one teaspoonful every five minutes and slowly increase the amount. Once full feeding amounts are reached and the infant has gone eight hours without vomiting, return to regular feeding.

For severe nausea, the prescription Phenergan (promethazine) may be given either as a suppository, liquid, or shot. For nausea that accompanies surgery or chemotherapy, Zofran (ondansetron) or Kytril (granisetron) stops the nausea impulse very effectively.

PINK EYE

A diagnosis of pink eye can be confusing as pink eye is a form of conjunctivitis, of which there are several different types: allergic, viral, and bacterial. The allergic class of conjunctivitis is caused by pet dander, mold spores, and pollen in the air, which in some can cause the eyes to begin to water and itch (see Allergic Conjunctivitis, pg. 133). Then the membrane covering the eyeball and the inner eyelid, also called the conjunctiva, becomes inflamed.

Viral conjunctivitis causes watery eyes and a thinner mucus discharge. Antibiotics aren't effective against this form of eye infection. It is diagnosed when a discharge of yellow pus appears in the child's eye. The eye may appear glued together upon awakening. The whites of the eyes and inner eyelids look red and bloodshot. Pain, itching, and burning are also primary symptoms.

Bacterial infections require prescription antibiotic drops or ointments from the doctor for treatment. Both viral and bacterial conjunctivitis are highly contagious and can be spread easily from eye to eye and from person to person.

NATURAL CHOICES
Gently wiping the outside of the eyes with warm washcloths can be soothing, as well as beneficial in flushing out bacteria. You should be sure to wash your child's hands often and replace the washcloths with

each use. This will greatly decrease the opportunity for bacterial or viral reinfection.

OVER-THE-COUNTER PRODUCTS

Over-the-counter eyedrops aren't generally recommended for treating Pink Eye caused by a virus or bacteria, but may be helpful when only an allergy is involved. For the allergic conjunctivitis sufferers, a safe solution to use at home is an eye wash with dilute boric acid or saline. Use an eyecup to gently flush the eye. This serves to soothe the irritation. Unfortunately, this will not kill bacteria present, so a prescription antibiotic will be required for a diagnosis of bacterial conjunctivitis.

DOCTOR VISITS

When little hands are constantly rubbing fiercely itching eyes, it is possible to tear the delicate eye membranes and allow an infection to develop. With children, this can happen very quickly. For most cases of bacteria conjunctivitis, the doctor may prescribe an antibiotic/ steroid combination, like Cortisporin Ophthalmic (polymixin B, neomycin, hydrocortisone) to both fight infection and reduce redness and inflammation.

Putting eyedrops into a child's eyes can be a difficult and sometimes frustrating experience. Wasting the drops not only could prolong the condition you're treating, but prescription eyedrops can be *very* expensive.

Following are a few hints that should help:

■ First, wash your hands. It would amaze you how many bacteria are living just on the tip of your finger! You don't want to introduce more bacteria into your child's eye.

■ Tilt your child's head backward. Try to keep his chin higher than his eyes.

■ Use that freshly washed index finger to pull the lower eyelid away from the eye. See the nice little pouch that forms?

■ Aim the medicine for that pouch. Don't attempt to put the drops directly on the eyeball. That can be very scary and will cause the best of us to blink before that drop hits.

■ Use care not to touch the tip of the dropper to the eyelid.

■ Many eyedrops or ointments can cause blurry vision. This can last for some time after applying them, so inform your child that this may happen and help him to stay quiet until his vision clears.

POISON IVY

Whether the rash is from poison ivy, poison oak, or poison sumac, the result is the same. A redness and swelling of the skin begins the unpleasantness. Soon the intensely itchy rash sets in, followed closely by small, oozing blisters.

The culprit behind all of these rashes is the chemical urushiol. Urushiol is the potent oil found inside the leaves of plants from the poison ivy, oak, and sumac families. Living, dormant, and dead plants of the poison ivy, oak, and sumac family all contain urushiol. Clear or yellowish in color, this oil causes itching virtually on contact. Over 85 percent of people are so allergic to this oil that just a tiny brush with it can trigger an intense allergic reaction.

This oil causing the rash is sticky and will stay around on anything that touches it—on your gardening gloves, shoes, and clothes, and even in the air if you are burning the pesky plants. Children coming into contact with these are at as much risk as if they had touched the plants themselves.

Often your child won't start itching right away, even if she's been exposed to the oil directly. It can take from a few hours to up to one week for a full-blown allergic reaction to be seen. Typically the first exposure to urushiol takes the longest time to develop into a rash. This is because the body is mounting a defense against what it sees as a foreign substance that must be removed at all costs. Second or third exposures can start itching within hours because the body now has antibodies present. The rash typically runs its full course in 14 to 20 days. That's a very long time for your little one to be itching, oozing, and miserable.

NATURAL CHOICES

Long sleeves and long pants may provide some protection when contact with the plants is unavoidable, but the best way of preventing a rash is to teach your child to identify and avoid the plants.

Identifiers for these itchy plants are:

■ We all know the adage "leaflets three, let it be" for poison ivy, which typically has glossier leaves with a distinctive three-leaflet pattern.

■ Poison oak can appear as a low shrub or a vine and can have leaves of different shapes, sizes, and colors depending on where it is growing.

■ Poison sumac grows in moist areas and resembles a small tree. Its branches can have seven to eight leaflets on each stem.

For situations when you're not 100 percent sure if there has been an exposure to poison ivy, oak, sumac, or any other itchy plant, simply wash the area with water as soon as possible. Soap and water is best, but use plain water if there is no soap available. Take as long as necessary and at least five minutes, keeping in mind that you are washing off an oil that is very sticky and determined to stay put.

OVER-THE-COUNTER PRODUCTS

For family camping trips and those times when possible exposure to poison ivy, poison oak, or poison sumac is unavoidable, try Ivy Block (bentoquatam). This is a product that will actually protect your child from exposure to poison ivy. It is applied to the skin and forms a barrier between the skin and urushiol; when the urushiol touches the Ivy Block, it can't reach the skin and cause a reaction. If your child is severely allergic, she may still get some minor itching, but nothing like what would happen without the Ivy Block.

Other over-the-counter products that focus on making the symptoms of poison ivy more bearable include:

■ Isopropyl rubbing alcohol is very effective for neutralizing the urushiol oil before the rash appears. Simply rub the affected areas of skin if contact with urushiol is suspected.

■ For an all-over body relief, you can try an Aveeno bath. The oatmeal bath soothes the skin and eases the itchiness. Use care to keep the water lukewarm to cool, as hot water makes the itching more severe.

■ If the itching becomes too intense, Benadryl (diphenhydramine) is an antihistamine that your child can take internally to make her more comfortable.

■ General body aches and pains from this battle your child's body is fighting can be treated with pain relievers, like Tylenol (acetaminophen).

■ Calamine Aerosol Spray by Band-Aid is a good choice for children over the age of two. Not only do you not have to touch the itchy, blistered skin, but this product also acts as a numbing anti-itch, and drying agent for weepy rashes. It contains calamine, camphor, and benzocaine.

DOCTOR VISITS

Poison ivy, poison oak, or poison sumac rashes are rarely dangerous themselves and will run their course over two to three weeks. However, if the rash spreads to your child's eyes, face, mouth, or genital areas, it's time to call the doctor. Higher strength prescription steroid creams may be required to control the swelling, itching, and spread of the rash. Steroid liquids or shots, like prednisolone (Orapred) or Medrol (methylprednisolone), may be prescribed in severe cases for short-term use and can bring quick relief from the inflammation and itch.

RASHES

There are many different types of rashes. Rashes may be caused by contact dermatitis, or a contact with an allergic substance outside the body, or by a viral illnesses, such as chicken pox or measles. Viral rashes may also accompany a cold, a cough, or a bout of diarrhea and are more common in babies and young children than in adults. Most rashes caused by viruses are not serious and usually disappear on their own over a few days to a week.

Contact dermatitis is usually very easy to identify because once the offending substance, such as urushiol, chemicals from laundry detergents, lotions, and so on, touches the skin, the redness, swelling, small blisters, and itching begin. This type of rash can be caused by what the body considers an allergen: irritating laundry soap, poison ivy, poison oak, grass, lotions, creams, even the dyes used to color clothes. Once the offending substance that causes the rash is removed, the rash generally goes away in a few days.

In rare cases, a rash is an early sign of a severe allergic reaction to a substance such as food, medication, or insect venom. The reaction may cause a life-threatening emergency if airways close or the body goes into shock (see Anaphylactic Shock, pg. 138.)

NATURAL CHOICES

A contact dermatitis rash can be cured quickly once the agent causing the irritation is removed. Unfortunately, sometimes it can take a bit of detective work to determine exactly what is causing the rash. This is especially true if your child has been exposed to the substance before without a reaction. The location of the rash may give good clues as to where, or what substance, it is coming from. Rashes on the torso may be related to a new detergent or fabric softener. Those around the head and ears may indicate a reaction to a new shampoo.

If you notice the beginning of what could be a contact dermatitis rash, it is a good idea to wash the area thoroughly with a mild soap and water. However, this can be dangerous if you're not sure whether the soap is to blame for the rash. Use soap that you're very familiar with or avoid the soap entirely and use cool water and moist cloths for easing the itch. A half-cup of cornstarch in tepid bathwater can also bring quick, temporary relief for the itchy child.

Keeping your child's fingernails clean and short helps avoid broken skin, which can lead to infection.

OVER-THE-COUNTER PRODUCTS

For contact rashes, the task is to stop the itch and to prevent skin infections. Making the child as comfortable as possible during the time the rash runs its course can be done with over-the-counter products. Over-the-counter hydrocortisone creams and ointments should be first in line when the itching starts. These are available in strengths from 0.5 to 1 percent. Apply every two hours until the rash feels less itchy and then four times a day until the itch is gone.

Benadryl Children's Allergy Relief (diphenhydramine) stops the itch from the inside. Favorite flavors of cherry and bubblegum make the medicine easier to swallow for little taste buds.

Band-Aid Calamine Aerosol Spray (calamine, camphor, and benzocaine) is a good choice for children over the age of two. The cool spray prevents you from having to touch their itchy, blistered skin. It also acts as a numbing anti-itch, and drying agent for weepy rashes.

DOCTOR VISITS

Rashes will typically go away on their own, but if the child has a temperature or the rash becomes severe, a doctor's visit is in order. Depending on the child's age, prescription steroid medicines like prednisone or prednisolone (Orapred) may be given for a short course to stop the inflammation.

If it isn't possible to determine the cause of the rash quickly, your child's doctor may do a patch test. This test places a variety of common irritants directly on small areas of the skin to see if a rash or irritation develops. If a rash develops under the patch, the doctor has identified the irritant as one to which the child is allergic. Now the focus can be on avoiding the offending irritant.

REYE'S SYNDROME

Reye's syndrome is very rare, with less than 20 cases each year in the United States, but it is a serious disease that can develop in children and teens under age 20. It occurs most often in children aged six to 12 years old. With Reye's syndrome, inflammation and swelling of the brain and liver occurs, with possible later damage to both organ systems.

Over-the-counter medications containing aspirin must carry the warning to avoid giving this product to anyone under the age of 15 who is experiencing an illness accompanied by a fever. The chicken pox and influenza virus carry special risk. Current thought is that the disease is brought on from a viral particle reaction with something in the chemical makeup of aspirin. This reaction produces a compound that the body perceives as deadly. The brain becomes inflamed and swells and the liver becomes overwhelmed by fats. Once the disease begins to progress, it moves quickly. Drowsiness, confusion, seizures, coma, and, in severe cases, death may result.

There is no cure for Reye's syndrome. The goal of treatment is to stop the brain and liver damage and prevent complications. All children with Reye's syndrome are treated in a hospital intensive care unit.

The first symptoms of Reye's syndrome appear four to seven days after the original viral illness begins. Symptoms are nausea, vomiting, and changes in mental function, including grogginess, disorientation, or confusion. Disorientation occurs because the child's liver isn't capable of filtering the high levels of ammonia that quickly build up. Eventually, the child may become delirious and slip into a coma.

NATURAL CHOICES

As a parent, there are ways you can help decrease the chances your child will develop Reye's syndrome. Because there is a strong link between the use of aspirin in children and the development of Reye's syndrome, do not give aspirin or products that contain aspirin to anyone younger than 20 years of age to treat an illness that causes a fever unless directed by a health professional. This is especially important if the child has chicken pox (varicella) or the flu (influenza).

Self-treatment is not recommended for Reye's syndrome. If severe nausea, vomiting, and disorientation occur, seek medical care immediately, even if your child has not had a recent viral infection or taken aspirin. Early medical treatment decreases the risk of long-term complications and death.

OVER-THE-COUNTER PRODUCTS

Over-the-counter medications are *not* recommended for self-treatment of Reye's syndrome. Use Tylenol (acetaminophen) or Motrin (ibuprofen) for children's pain and fever relief. Use care when choosing over-the-counter medicines for your family. Aspirin is found in many nonprescription medicines and may sneak into your medicine chest.

Read labels carefully before giving a nonprescription medication to your child. Beware of hidden aspirin. Some medicines containing aspirin (or salicylates related to aspirin) that you might not be aware of are: Pepto-Bismol, Excedrin, and Alka-Seltzer. Aspirin is also called by the following names:

- Acetyl salicylate

- Acetylsalicylic acid

- Salicylic acid

- Salicylate or subsalicylate

DOCTOR VISITS

If your child is recovering from a viral illness and suddenly develops severe nausea, vomiting, or behavioral changes, call the doctor right away. The symptoms of Reye's syndrome are similar to those of many other childhood conditions, so when a child is brought in with a suspected case, a liver biopsy and spinal tap are often done to confirm that the child's condition is indeed Reye's syndrome and not something else entirely.

Medical treatment of Reye's syndrome consists of supporting the child's heart, lung, and brain functions while keeping blood levels of ammonia low until the symptoms disappear. For cases when the brain begins to swell, steroids may be given. If the disease is diagnosed early, most children recover from Reye's syndrome in a few weeks.

RINGWORM

Ringworm isn't caused by a worm, it's caused by a fungus. Ringworm gets its name from the round shape of the infection, with small bumps that look like blisters around the edges. You'll also hear ringworm of the skin referred to as tinea corporis. The same fungus responsible for ringworm also causes athlete's foot and jock itch. Ringworm is common in children and may be spread by contact with animals or outdoor areas where the fungus lives. Moist areas on the body provide a haven for the fungus to thrive.

The rash is often very itchy and can spread on the body quickly. It is important to treat ringworm as soon as possible, because the full course of treatment may take several weeks to complete. With children, there is a high risk of secondary bacterial infections from open areas of the skin caused by scratching.

NATURAL CHOICES

Pets living in the home can be a source of the ringworm fungus. If it has patches of missing hair or scaly, dry skin—signs of a fungal infection—bring your pet to the veterinarian for treatment.

Keep your child's skin clean and dry and let them wear loose-fitting cotton clothing. Always dry your child completely after baths. After drying her skin with a towel, allow her skin to air dry before putting clothes on. If someone in the family has ringworm, wash all clothes, towels, and sheets in hot water with laundry detergent.

Keeping the child's fingernails clipped short and kept clean should help decrease the chance of an infection from broken skin.

While your child is being treated for ringworm, she should avoid activity areas where she may spread the infection to others, such as gyms, wrestling matches, or swimming pools.

OVER-THE-COUNTER PRODUCTS

If your child has ringworm, use a nonprescription antifungal, like Micatin, Tinactin, Lamisil, or Lotrimin. These contain miconazole, terbinafine, or clotrimazole as their active ingredients and come in cream, powder, liquid, and spray forms. So which is better?

■ Powders are good for places where sweating is a problem, like in the folds of skin or where clothing is in constant contact with the skin.

■ Sprays are the easiest to apply, but may be cold and may waste medicine unless you have great aim. Check appropriate ages on the products before using on your child's skin.

■ Creams or lotions can be applied directly to the rash and are generally thought to be the most effective. Wash the rash with soap and water, remove any pieces of dried skin, and spread an antifungal cream over the rash. Apply the cream beyond the edge or border of the rash.

Lamisil AT (terbinafine) in the cream form is a convenient and effective way to treat ringworm for children 12 years and older. Wash the affected skin with soap and water and dry completely before applying. Spray the affected area once a day (morning or night) for one week or as directed by a doctor. Don't have your child stop taking the medication just because his symptoms go away. If the symptoms do not improve after two weeks, call the doctor.

Children's Benadryl (diphenhydramine) can help decrease the itch from the inside. If the itching becomes severe, applying a light coating of hydrocortisone cream or ointment to the rash should help quite a bit.

DOCTOR VISITS

If you're uncertain about whether your child's rash is ringworm or not, bring them into the doctor for diagnosis. Certain types of ringworm will appear fluorescent if the skin is examined in a darkened room with a blue light called a Wood's lamp. A more definitive diagnosis can be made by scraping the affected area of skin and examining the cells under a microscope.

ROSEOLA

Roseola is a viral condition characterized by a high fever lasting three to seven days, followed by a bright red rash on the child's trunk, arms, legs, neck, and face. Fighting a fever is tough under the best of circumstances, but when your little one breaks out in a rash just when you think the trouble is over, that's enough to worry any parent. After four to five days of a high fever, the rash appears. By this time, the fever is either completely gone or has dropped. Typically, the rash isn't itchy or scaly and only lasts from a few hours to two days.

This virus is most often seen in children from six months of age to one year, but can occur anywhere in the three-month to four-year-old range. It is easily spread through saliva or the fecal/oral route with an incubation period of five to 15 days. Because a virus causes roseola, antibiotics aren't effective.

The real concern with roseola is the possibility of febrile convulsions (see Febrile Seizures, pg. 219) from the high fever. Temperatures can rise as high as 105° F and should be brought down as quickly as possible. Other symptoms may include a runny nose and sore throat.

NATURAL CHOICES
Cool baths and cool clothes help the feverish body to feel better. This disease is contagious, so keeping your little one away from others is important until the rash has disappeared.

OVER-THE-COUNTER PRODUCTS
Fortunately, fevers from roseola usually respond quickly to children's acetaminophen products, like Tylenol. For the little ones, use the infant drops. Older children usually prefer the chewable tablets in

cherry or grape flavor. Motrin (ibuprofen), in the corresponding dose for your child's weight and age, can help bring down fever and make them feel more comfortable.

DOCTOR VISITS

Because this condition is difficult to distinguish from others with high fever symptoms, like urinary tract infections or measles, it is important to have the child checked by the doctor. If there are any questions as to the type of condition, the doctor may order a blood test.

RUNNY NOSE (RHINITIS)

Whether it's from an allergy or a cold, a child's runny nose is not a pleasant thing. You wipe, they wipe, and all you have is more wiping and a red, irritated little nose. The first step is to determine what is causing the problem.

If it is caused by an allergy, the runny nose generally comes around seasonally, especially if the allergy is pollen related. It may also appear whenever the kitty or puppy comes over to play if it is caused by pet dander. You can generally assume allergies if, along with a runny nose, your child has red and watery eyes. The drainage from a runny nose caused by allergies is usually clear and thin, but may become thicker and cloudy or yellowish if a nasal or sinus infection develops. (See Allergies, pg. 236). With a cold, the child may have a slight fever and cough along with the runny nose. Or the nose may alternate between runny and stuffed. A cold generally only lasts for one to two weeks. (See Colds, pg. 180).

Whatever the cause, drying up the child's nose is a priority. Antihistamines do the job well if your child has a cold or an allergy. Avoid decongestants with allergies because they can make the dripping worse.

NATURAL CHOICES

Runny noses serve a purpose: nasal mucus and discharge wash viruses, bacteria, and allergens out of the nose and sinuses. Usually blowing the nose is all that's needed. Apply petroleum jelly to cleaned areas outside of the nose openings to protect them from irritation. Using soft tissues with lotion added is helpful for extremely sore noses.

OVER-THE-COUNTER PRODUCTS

Antihistamines, like Benadryl liquid and chewables (diphenhydramine), have been the "runny nose driers" for many years. Many doctors still recommend this as the top over-the-counter product for controlling cold and allergy symptoms, like a runny nose. However, newer nonsedating antihistamines, like Claritin (loratidine), are now available without a prescription for use in children. The liquid and quick-dissolving Reditabs work well for children over six years old. The bedtime dosage is especially important for allowing sleep and time to heal the lining of the nose.

DOCTOR VISITS

Usually just describing your child's symptoms to the doctor results in a correct diagnosis for allergies, but if the child has trouble breathing or unusual redness around the eyes, it's time for a visit to the pediatrician.

Unfortunately, if it's a cold affecting your child's nose, it will simply have to run its course. Antibiotics aren't effective against the cold virus.

For long-term allergy relief, the physician might recommend a series of allergy shots to allow the child's body to build up immunity against allergens he might come into contact with on a regular basis.

Seasonal allergies may require prescription medicines for the older child. Nasal steroids, like Nasacort AQ (triamcinolone) or Beconase AQ (beclomethasone), help to decrease swelling of nasal membranes and make breathing easier.

SCABIES

Scabies are one of the conditions parents hope never comes into contact with their family members. Scabies are tiny (0.4mm) mites with four pairs of legs who tunnel under the skin and lay their eggs. The eggs hatch within two weeks and the baby mites make their way out again. Unfortunately, this is a common skin infection that is typically spread by close contact with an infested person. It is also possible for mites to spread via shared personal belongings, such as towels and linens. The mites prefer the webs of fingers, wrists, elbows, armpits, and groin area. Scabies infestation appears as short, dark, wavy lines on the skin surface.

Scabies can be spread during the entire time a person is infested, even during the weeks before symptoms appear. It commonly affects several family members during the same period of time. During a first exposure, the family may not show symptoms for two to six weeks after being bug-ridden. Then the itching begins. Small, itchy blisters appear when the skin is scratched or just after a bath. Secondary infections occur when the skin is torn open from the intense itching.

Bacteria find a home in the broken skin and often a prescription antibiotic is required.

NATURAL CHOICES

Close personal contact spreads scabies, so the only way to avoid infestation is to avoid exposure. Limit contact between other family members and the affected child's clothing, towels, toys, and bedding to avoid the spread of scabies.

Sometimes the source of the mite can be traced to an area of the backyard or a favorite swimming hole. Once identified, these areas must be avoided in order to prevent a recurrence.

OVER-THE-COUNTER PRODUCTS

Scabies does not go away on its own. Unfortunately, a prescription treatment is necessary to cure scabies; the scabies mite is resistant to nonprescription-strength medications. Some itching may continue several weeks after a successful treatment due to dead mites and tunnels still in the skin. For over-the-counter itch relief, an antihistamine like Benadryl (diphenhydramine) may be effective for short-term relief.

DOCTOR VISITS

Your doctor may be able to diagnose scabies based on your child's symptoms and those of people your child has close contact with. Your doctor may gently scrape some skin from the affected area and examine it for signs of mites under a microscope.

After a diagnosis is made, the doctor will likely prescribe a medicated topical cream called Elimite (permethrin). The first step to control a scabies infestation usually involves softening the skin with soap and water to make sure the pesticide treatments can penetrate well. An evening bath followed by overnight treatment works best. Then the medicine is applied from the neck down to cover the whole body—that's the whole body, from the neck to the soles of the feet. This cream is left on for at least eight hours. Overnight is good. Then wash it off thoroughly. There may be some residual itching for a day or two. If it doesn't go away, a second treatment may be required. Check with the doctor before using a second application.

A newer medication is available in pill form that may be prescribed for resistant scabies. Stromectal (ivermectin) is taken in one dose followed by another two weeks later. Sometimes Stromectal (ivermectin) is combined with permethrin (Elimite) cream for treating scabies. Current studies have not been done on children under 35 pounds.

SORE THROAT

There are actually many causes of children's sore throats. Bacteria or viruses can cause an infectious sore throat. Postnasal drip from an allergy can bring on a miserable irritation to the back of the throat. Shouting all afternoon at the soccer game or being exposed to excessive smoke may also bring on throat pain in youngsters. Your child can develop a dry sore throat from breathing in cold air through his mouth during cold winter months.

Only ten percent of children's sore throats can be treated with antibiotics. This is because most sore throats are caused by a virus. A host of viruses, called upper respiratory viruses, are responsible for a majority of the sore throats experienced every year during cough and cold season. The Epstein-Barr virus gives us the sore throats from infectious mononucleosis or mono. Coxsackie virus brings on a sore throat accompanied by small blisters around the back of the throat.

The type of sore throat most commonly caused by bacteria is called strep throat. Strep throat can occur at any age, but is most common in children ages three to 15. The most common symptoms of a strep throat infection are sudden, severe sore throat, pain or difficulty swallowing, fever over 101° F, swollen tonsils and lymph nodes, and white or yellow spots on the back of a bright red throat (see Strep Throat, pg. 295).

It is important to take a sore throat seriously. Left untreated, a child's sore throat can progress to a more serious condition, called rheumatic fever, where the heart valves are damaged. Another worry is glomerulonephritis, a bacterial infection beginning in the throat that may find a home in the kidneys where more damage can be done.

NATURAL CHOICES

Sore throats generally run their course within a few days. In the meantime, you can help make the child as comfortable as possible by taking the following steps:

■ Use a steam mist vaporizer to keep throat tissues moist while your child is sleeping.

■ Change the family's toothbrushes every month to toss harmful bacteria out and prevent sore throats from recurring.

■ If your child's doctor has ruled out a bacterial infection, the best at-home treatment is to keep the throat moist. Have your child drink plenty of water. Sucking on ice chips can also soothe and numb sore throats.

■ Have your child gargle with warm salt water to help reduce swelling. Orange juice may be high in vitamin C, but it may also sting irritated throats.

■ Place warm towels or cloths directly on your child's neck, which can also help alleviate some of the pain and swelling associated with a sore throat.

OVER-THE-COUNTER PRODUCTS

For children over the age of three, try the Cepacol Maximum Strength Sore Throat Spray in honey lemon flavor. You spray this directly on your child's aching and burning throat and have them swallow. Within seconds, there is no more pain. It uses the numbing agent dyclonine hydrochloride to provide fast, temporary relief for sore throat and mouth pain.

For children over the age of five, lozenges, like cough drops or hard candy, that contain numbing agents, like benzocaine, can help temporarily reduce the pain. Cepacol Citrus lozenges contain two anesthetics, menthol and benzocaine, to relieve the pain of swallowing with a sore throat.

Pain relievers, like children's Tylenol (acetaminophen) or Motrin (ibuprofen), are effective for the body aches and pains that accompany a sore throat. These also help to bring down the swelling and inflammation of sore throats associated with the common cold.

DOCTOR VISITS

Because so many different things can cause a sore throat, it's a good idea to get your child checked by the doctor at the first sign of trouble, especially if he has a fever higher than 101° F. The doctor will take a visual examination and may also order a throat culture, which can usually be read in the office. The doctor is looking for the presence of bacteria, usually from the strep family. Strep can be fought with a course of antibiotics, like amoxicillin or Augmentin. If your child's doctor does prescribe an antibiotic, remember to give it to the child exactly as directed. This means you should finish the entire five-, ten-, or 14-day therapy until the liquid or tablets are finished. It is important to finish the medication completely even if the sore throat feels better. Your child's body is still fighting the bacteria, so give it all the help you can.

However, with most sore throats, especially those caused by viruses, there is no magic bullet. Keeping the child comfortable will be the prescription.

STREP THROAT

Strep throat is an infection of the pharynx, which is the part of the throat between the tonsils and the larynx. It is also called acute streptococcal pharyngitis. When your child's doctor takes a culture of the back of the child's throat with a swab, she's looking for presence of the *Streptococcus pyogenes* bacterium, which is responsible for about ten percent of sore throats. The type of strep that most commonly infects the throat is called group A beta-hemolytic streptococcus (GABS). Other types that can sometimes infect the throat are groups C and G strep bacteria.

Strep throat occurs most commonly from October to April, and most often in children three to 15 years old. The most common symptoms of a strep throat infection are sudden, severe sore throat, pain or difficulty swallowing, fever over 101° F, swollen tonsils and lymph nodes, and white or yellow spots on the back of a bright red throat.

Strep throat is more serious than your average sore throat and tends to last a little longer. Prescription antibiotics are recommended to prevent the bacteria from entering the heart and causing the complication of rheumatic fever.

NATURAL CHOICES

Little ones can benefit from a steam mist vaporizer to keep throat tissues moist while they're sleeping. Rest is essential to give the body time to fight the infection. Changing the family's toothbrushes every month can also toss out harmful bacteria and prevent sore throats from recurring. Strep throat is very contagious, so limit sharing of cups and drinks between the infected child and other family members.

As with other sore throats, drinking plenty of water is a good idea to keep the throat moist and help flush out harmful bacteria. Gargling with warm salt water can help reduce throat swelling and ease the pain. Orange juice may be high in vitamin C, but it may also sting irritated throats, so look to less acidic juices, like apple or grape. Warm towels or cloths placed directly on the neck can also help decrease the pain and swelling associated with strep throat.

OVER-THE-COUNTER PRODUCTS

For children over the age of three, try the Cepacol Maximum Strength Sore Throat Spray in honey lemon flavor. You spray this directly on your child's aching and burning throat and have them swallow. Within seconds, there is no more pain. It uses the numbing agent dyclonine hydrochloride to provide fast, temporary relief for sore throat and mouth pain.

For children over the age of five, lozenges, like cough drops or hard candy, that contain numbing agents, like benzocaine, can help temporarily reduce the pain. Cepacol Citrus lozenges contain two anesthetics, menthol and benzocaine, to relieve the pain of swallowing with a sore throat.

Pain relievers, like children's acetaminophen (Tylenol) or ibuprofen (Motrin), are effective for the body aches and pains that accompany strep throat. These help to bring down the swelling and inflammation of tissue in the back of the throat.

DOCTOR VISITS

Because so many different things can cause a sore throat, it's a good idea to get your child checked by the doctor at the first sign of trouble, especially if he has a fever higher than 101° F. The doctor will take a visual examination and may also order a rapid strep test, which can usually be read in the office. Strep can be fought with a course of antibiotics, like amoxicillin or Augmentin. If your child's doctor does prescribe an antibiotic, remember to give it to the child exactly as directed. This means the child should finish the entire five-, ten-, or 14-day therapy until the liquid or tablets are finished. It is important that the child finishes the medication completely even if the sore throat feels better. Your child's body is still fighting the bacteria, so give it all the help you can. Antibiotics will prevent rheumatic fever even if started up to nine days after the first symptoms of strep throat.

Antibiotics are typically prescribed for children who have:

■ A positive rapid strep test or positive throat culture.

■ Three of the four following signs or symptoms: a recent fever, white or yellow spots coating the throat and/or tonsils, swollen or tender lymph nodes on the neck, or an absence of other cold and cough symptoms.

■ Recent exposure to strep or to someone who has had rheumatic fever. In these cases, preventive (prophylactic) antibiotics may be given.

■ Several family members with repeated strep infections as confirmed by positive throat cultures.

SWIMMER'S EAR

Swimmer's ear, or otitis externa, is caused by bacteria and fungal infections from the accumulation of water, sand, or other debris that becomes trapped deep in the ear canal. Frequent swimming or showering can strip the normal lining of the ear canal and allow bacterial or fungal growth in the trapped water pockets. The ear canal closes from earwax accumulation or swelling of the Eustachian tubes and the infection persists.

Symptoms of an ear canal inflammation include a feeling of fullness in the ear, itching, pain, discharge, or hearing loss. Persistent ringing or sloshing in the ear is also felt with this type of infection.

Unlike a middle ear infection, the pain of swimmer's ear is worse with chewing, pressing on the "tag" in front of the ear, or wiggling the earlobe. A more advanced case with inflammation or infection often clears up with antibiotics, and most cases of swimmer's ear can be prevented with home treatment.

NATURAL CHOICES

Ask your pharmacist for a small dropper bottle. Add a 50/50 mixture of isopropyl alcohol and white vinegar. Use one to three drops in the ears after swimming or showering to evaporate the excess water. The vinegar covers the ear canal and lowers the pH. Bacteria and fungus don't grow as well in low-pH areas. Parents have used this home remedy for years to dry out the ear canals of little swimmers susceptible to swimmer's ear.

OVER-THE-COUNTER PRODUCTS

Once the original infection has been cleared with prescription antibiotics, use solutions like Auro-Dri and Swim-Ear (isopropyl alcohol) to dry ear canals by removing excess water. The alcohol mixes with trapped water and evaporates quickly, stopping the growth of bacteria and fungus.

Star-Otic uses acetic acid, boric acid, and Burow's solution (aluminum acetate) to keep the ear canal highly acidic so an infection can't find a home. Propylene glycol is another important ingredient in Star-Otic that acts as a drying agent. Use three to five drops before and after swimming and bathing. Stop using the drops if any additional irritation occurs.

DOCTOR VISITS

While many cases of sloshing and fullness of swimmer's ear can be treated with over-the-counter products, there are certain things to look for that warrant a visit to the doctor:

- Your child's ear pain and itching persist or get worse after three days of home treatment.

- The ear canal, the opening to the ear canal, the external ear, or the skin around the external ear becomes swollen, red, or very painful.

- Your child develops foul-smelling discharge from the ear that does not appear to be earwax.

- Your child's ear symptoms are accompanied by a fever of 100° F or higher.

■ Your child develops dizziness or unsteadiness.

■ Your child's ear discomfort lasts for longer than two weeks.

■ Your child's symptoms become more severe or frequent.

The doctor may prescribe an antibiotic to be taken orally—commonly amoxicillin—or one that is put directly in the ear—commonly Floxin. Anti-inflammatory eardrops, like Voltaren, are available for swelling, and pain-relieving medicines, like Auralgan, are often prescribed to be used in the ear.

Some tips for getting more medicine into the ears than on your child's clothes are:

■ First, warm the drops to body temperature by rolling the container in your hands or placing it in a cup of warm water for a few minutes. Inserting cold eardrops can cause pain and dizziness.

■ Have the child lie down, ear facing up.

■ Place one or two drops on the wall of the ear canal so air can escape and drops can get into the ear. Gently wiggling the outer ear will help.

■ You may find it easier to insert eardrops in a small child's ear by holding the child on your lap with his or her legs around your waist and head down on your knees. If possible, remain in this position for two to three minutes.

TEETHING

The first three years of your baby's life are quite busy. From the dental standpoint alone, the baby will cut 20 new teeth! The lower and upper incisors (front teeth) are the first to make an appearance, usually from just after birth to one year of age. This can be a painful time for those tender young gums.

Symptoms of teething include drooling, an inability to sleep and fussiness, chewing on anything they can put into their little mouths, swollen gums, and a poor appetite. Be on the lookout for erupting teeth, as they can be felt a few days before they break the gum surface.

NATURAL CHOICES

Comfort is key during the painful period while the teeth are ready to break the surface. Here are some helpful hints for helping your baby manage the pain:

- Use clean washcloths soaked in cold water as chew toys.

- Put teething rings into the refrigerator for a short time before use, which will cool and ease the pain.

- Use hard teething biscuits as gum soothers.

- Swab tender gums with a soft cloth or soft bristle toothbrush to teach good dental habits.

Homeopathic remedies have been shown to relieve fussiness and the discomfort of teething. Names to look for are Hyland's Teething Tablets, Humphrey's "3," and Hyland's Teething Gel.

OVER-THE-COUNTER PRODUCTS

Medicines applied directly to the gums provide instant relief for sore gums. These contain the numbing agent benzocaine as the active ingredient in strengths from seven to ten percent. Names to look for include Baby Oragel, Zilactin Baby, or Baby Anbesol. These are applied directly to the gums on the area of the emerging tooth, not more than four times a day, and only for babies over four months old unless otherwise directed by the pediatrician.

Infant's Motrin Drops are approved by the Food and Drug Administration for pain relief in teething infants to six months of age. The medicine reduces swelling and inflammation. The eight-hour dose is 50mg (1.25ml dropper) for babies 12 to 17 pounds and 75mg (1.5ml dropper) for babies 18 to 23 pounds. With the little ones, it is important to only use the enclosed dropper to measure the dose. Shake the medicine well. Be aware of ibuprofen medication allergies, which appear as hives, swelling of the face, and difficulty breathing (wheezing).

DOCTOR VISITS

Teething doesn't usually require prescription medications. However, if your baby's temperature spikes over 101° F and she seems unusually fussy and uncomfortable, bring her in to visit the doctor. You'll probably be told that everything is just fine, but it's better to be sure.

TINNITUS

Tinnitus, or ringing in the ears, can be an especially worrisome problem for older children. Tinnitus is defined as a noise in the ear that can only be heard by the person experiencing it. The sound can be described as buzzing, ringing, chirping, roaring, whistling, or even hissing. However, with children, it is often described as a "funny" sound, or a younger child may simply lack the vocabulary to describe the sounds in his head.

This condition can be caused by swelling in the ear canal, exposure to loud noises, head injury, chronic ear infections, physical ear blockage (see Earwax, pg. 211), or a reaction to certain medicines, like aspirin, quinidine, and quinine. Tinnitus may also be one of the first signs of a more serious medical condition, like high blood pressure and low thyroid, so it's important to let your child's doctor take a look if your child frequently complains of this problem.

Caregivers should be alert to signs of tinnitus that may appear as behavior problems, including poor attention and concentration, depression, insomnia, restlessness, and lack of focus.

NATURAL CHOICES
Limit caffeine consumption, as this tends to make tinnitus worse. If insomnia develops because of this condition, the use of a "white noise" machine or soft music playing by the child's bedside might prove helpful.

OVER-THE-COUNTER PRODUCTS
While there are no specific over-the-counter products for the treatment of tinnitus, it has been shown that aspirin and aspirin-containing products can make it worse. Some medicines containing aspirin (or salicylates related to aspirin) that you might not be aware of are Pepto-Bismol, Excedrin, and Alka-Seltzer. Aspirin is also called by the following names:

- Acetyl salicylate

- Acetylsalicylic acid

- Salicylic acid

- Salicylate or subsalicylate

It is important that *no* aspirin or aspirin-containing products be given to children under the age of 15 to treat illnesses with a fever due to the risk of Reye's syndrome (see Reye's Syndrome, pg. 282).

DOCTOR VISITS

If you suspect tinnitus might be a problem, a thorough evaluation by a specialist is in order, and most often you will need a referral from your pediatrician or primary care physician. Depending on the age and abilities of the child, different tests will be performed to judge the degree and severity of the condition. Several sessions may be required to complete the tests.

Your child's doctor may fit him with a special hearing aid that masks the tinnitus sounds and makes hearing clearer. Another therapy is auditory habituation. Here a small device plays a white noise that is lower in volume than the tinnitus noise, so the brain learns to ignore the tinnitus. This has been shown to be a very effective permanent treatment.

URINARY TRACT INFECTIONS

Urinary tract infections (UTIs) occur in an estimated three percent of girls and one percent of boys by the age of 11. Some researchers believe these estimates are low because many cases of UTI go undetected. The symptoms are not always obvious to parents, and younger children are usually unable to describe how they feel. Recognizing and treating UTIs is important. With infants, UTIs can be a sign of urinary reflux. Untreated UTIs can lead to serious kidney problems that could threaten the life of your child.

Symptoms of a UTI vary with the age of the child. She may have only a low-grade fever, experience nausea and vomiting, or just not seem to feel well. Other symptoms include pain in the abdomen and pelvic area, frequent urination, painful urination, cloudy or unusual-smelling urine, or pain under the side of the rib cage or in the lower back.

Normal urine is sterile, which means it contains no bacteria naturally. Bacteria may, at times, get into the urinary tract (and the urine) from the skin around the genital/rectal area by traveling up to the bladder through the tubes called urethras. When this happens, the bacteria can infect and inflame the bladder, resulting in swelling and pain in the lower abdomen and side. Another name for this condition is cystitis. If the bacteria travel farther up to the kidneys, an infection can develop. The infection is usually accompanied by pain and fever. Kidney infections are much more serious than bladder infections, so prompt medical attention is required if a UTI is suspected.

NATURAL CHOICES

Offer lots of water, along with cranberry juice, especially during the first 24 hours after your child has started antibiotic treatment. This will help make the urine less concentrated and wash out the bacteria causing infection.

Some experts feel that the harsh detergents in some bubble baths may irritate the genital area and urethra of little girls, making them more susceptible to UTIs. If your daughter is prone to UTIs, try cutting back on the bubble baths to see if that helps.

OVER-THE-COUNTER PRODUCTS

There are no recommended over-the-counter treatments for UTIs in children. Prompt medical attention is required to prevent the infection from spreading to the kidneys.

DOCTOR VISITS

If your child experiences any of these symptoms, call the doctor right away. A UTI can be easily treated with antibiotics, but a kidney infection may cause long-term damage to your child.

■ An unusual smell or color of urine on the diaper.

■ A high temperature and an appearance of sickness for more than a day without signs of a runny nose or other obvious symptoms of discomfort.

■ A discomfort urinating, often with pain or burning.

■ Lower back pain or pain under the rib cage.

The doctor will take a urinalysis by examining a urine specimen for white blood cells, blood, and bacteria. A clean-catch urine specimen is needed, meaning that the older child must carefully clean the opening to the urethra, begin urinating into the toilet, and then catch a bit of urine in a sterile cup for examination. For a younger child, the doctor may place a plastic collection bag over your child's genital area (sealed to the skin with an adhesive strip) if the child is not yet toilet trained.

If the diagnosis is a UTI, antibiotics, like Bactrim, are prescribed to kill the bacteria. After a few doses of the antibiotic, your child may appear much better, but often several days may pass before all symptoms are gone. In any case, your child should take the medicine for as long as the doctor says. Do not stop medications because the symptoms have gone away. Infections may return, and bacteria can resist future treatment if the drug is stopped too soon.

For older children, there are certain medications, like Pyridium (phenazopyridine hydrochloride,) that may be used to treat the burning sensation that accompanies a UTI.

WRESTLER'S HERPES

Who would have thought that adolescent wrestlers would have an entire strain of virus named after them? The offender here is the herpes simplex type 1 virus (HSV-1) in a condition commonly called herpes gladiatorum or wrestler's herpes. This condition is spread from rough, direct, skin-to-skin contact. It usually occurs on the jaw area or trunk and is spread from tight wrestling holds and locks.

Teen wrestlers and rugby players are most often seen with this condition. There are usually no other symptoms than the skin rash, but some teens may experience fever, swollen lymph nodes, sore throats, weakness, and eye infections.

Before physical symptoms appear, there may be burning or stinging at the infected site. The incubation period is two to 14 days. Small, raised groups of vesicles filled with fluid appear on a red, inflamed area of skin. The blister-like vesicles burst and the area is covered with small, hard scabs.

NATURAL CHOICES

Rules differ within each organization, but typically if there are vesicles and ulcers present on the skin, the wrestler is disqualified. This is to prevent the spread of the virus among all competitors. If the rash is scabbed and dry after at least five days of antibiotic treatment, the wrestler is considered noncontagious and may compete.

OVER-THE-COUNTER PRODUCTS

Due to the viral nature of this skin condition, there are no current over-the-counter products recommended for treatment of wrestler's herpes.

DOCTOR VISITS

The doctor can obtain a culture of the virus on the opening of the skin vesicles and put the cells in a viral medium to grow. A Tzanck smear will give faster results.

Medication prescribed for wrestler's herpes is usually a once-a-day dosage of 500mg Valtrex (valacyclovir). This antiviral is effective for preventing recurrences once the condition has been diagnosed. Zovirax (acyclovir) is another antiviral used for wrestler's herpes in a 200mg dose three times daily for ten days. These medicines are most effective when used in the early stages of the infection while the cells are rapidly dividing.

Family First-Aid Kit

- ❑ Ace bandage
- ❑ Adhesive bandages, in assorted sizes
- ❑ Gauze rolls and pads, in assorted sizes
- ❑ Adhesive tape (cloth), one-inch thickness
- ❑ Alcohol or antiseptic wound wipes
- ❑ Antiseptic/anesthetic spray, like Bactine
- ❑ Hydrogen peroxide, for cleaning cuts and scrapes
- ❑ Antibiotic ointment for cuts and scrapes
- ❑ Ibuprofen or similar anti-inflammatory pain-reliever tablets
- ❑ Burn cream or aloe vera–based gel for minor burns
- ❑ Insect bite/sting stick, like AfterBite
- ❑ Suncreen (do not use on babies younger than six months)
- ❑ Calamine lotion or hydrocortisone cream for itchy rashes
- ❑ Infant's and children's acetaminophen or ibuprofen, liquid or chewables, for use as recommended by your pediatrician
- ❑ Children's decongestant, for use as recommended by your pediatrician
- ❑ Ipecac syrup and activated charcoal for accidental poisonings, for use *only* after a recommendation by Poison Control
- ❑ Cotton balls and swabs
- ❑ Eye wash kit

- ❑ Antinausea/vomiting liquid Emetrol
- ❑ Instant cold pack
- ❑ Rubbing alcohol for cleaning thermometers
- ❑ Petroleum jelly (Vaseline)
- ❑ Scissors
- ❑ Smelling salts
- ❑ A rectal thermometer for infants and a digital thermometer for other family members
- ❑ Tweezers for removing splinters or ticks

ADDED EXTRAS

- ❑ CPR instruction card
- ❑ Disposable latex gloves
- ❑ EpiPen or similar epinepherine auto-injector for severe allergic reactions (see Anaphylactic Shock, pg. 138)
- ❑ First-aid guidebook
- ❑ Hand sanitzier (alcohol gel)
- ❑ Heating pad
- ❑ Wet wipes

MAKE SURE YOU . . .

- ❑ Check the expiration dates on all creams, ointments, and sprays.
- ❑ Throw away any product with an old expiration date or soon-to-expire date.
- ❑ Replenish supplies as they get low.
- ❑ Keep a card in the kit with all medicine allergies for each affected family member.

New Baby First-Aid Kit

With a new baby in the house, things may seem a little chaotic at times. Having a first-aid kit for the new baby will help you to focus on treating little problems when they occur, rather than scrambling around trying to find medicine that may have passed its expiration date or may not be suitable for young children.

Find a sturdy plastic container for home use that's large enough to hold necessary items and can grow with your child. A smaller kit for car and travel is also a good idea for busy parents.

Here are some essentials:

❑ Rectal thermometer

❑ Nasal aspirator bulb syringe and saline nasal drops

❑ Infant's formula liquid decongestant or antihistamine, for use as directed by your pediatrician

❑ Petroleum jelly (Vaseline); to lubricate a rectal thermometer

❑ Acetaminophen (Tylenol) and/or ibuprofen (Motrin, Advil) in infant formulas, to reduce fever and relieve pain. Include the dosing chart from the box (see Dosing and Administering Children's medicines pg. 59).

❑ Medicine dispenser. Most infant's and children's medications come with a measuring and dispensing tool and it's important to use that one. However, if the medicine doesn't come with a proper dosing instrument, ask your pharmacist for a syringe, spoon, dropper, and/or medicine cup to administer medicine to your child.

❑ Mild liquid soap or prepackaged baby-safe cleansing wipes, to clean minor scrapes

Check your first-aid kit every six months (or when the clocks jump ahead or back an hour) and replace any items that were used or have become outdated. As the baby gets older, add items to the Family's first-aid kit (see Family First-Aid Kit, pg. 309).

Keep a note card with current phone numbers and tape this information inside your kit. Keep another card in your purse or wallet, as well as by every telephone. Art supply stores carry inexpensive plastic laminate sheets; use these to ensure the numbers don't get blurry or smudged. Here are the numbers to keep:

■ Your health care provider, pharmacy, and nearest hospital.

■ Nearby relatives or neighbors who can provide immediate assistance, such as childcare for a sibling or a ride to the hospital.

■ The Poison Control Center

■ Local emergency services, if "911" is not available in your area.

■ Your own cell phone number and your own home phone number, along with your address and the nearest cross street, in case a babysitter or someone else makes an emergency call from your home.

Children's Health Resources

Listed below are a selection of useful health web sites, addresses, and phone numbers. All information is correct as of this writing. However, web sites and phone numbers may change.

ALLERGY AND ASTHMA
Allergy and Asthma Network/
Mothers of Asthmatics, Inc.
2751 Prosperity Avenue, Suite 150
Fairfax, VA 22031
800-878-4403; 703-641-9595
http://www.aanma.org

Asthma & Allergy Foundation of
America
1233 20th Street NW, Suite 402
Washington, DC 20036
800-7ASTHMA (800-727-8462);
202-466-7643
e-mail: info@aafa.org
http://www.aafa.org

ANEMIA
Cooley's Anemia Foundation
129-09 26th Avenue
Flushing, NY 11354
800-522-7222; 718-321-CURE
(718-321-2873)
http://www.thalassemia.org

ATTENTION DEFICIT DISORDER
Children and Adults with
Attention-Deficit/Hyperactivity
Disorder
8181 Professional Place, Suite 201
Landover, MD 20785
800-233-4050; 301-306-7070
http://www.chadd.org

National Attention Deficit Disorder
Association
1788 Second Street, Suite 200
Highland Park, IL 60035
847-432-ADDA (847-432-2332)
e-mail: mail@add.org
http://www.add.org

AUTISM
Autism Research Institute
4182 Adams Avenue
San Diego, CA 92116
619-281-7165
http://www.autism.com/ari

Autism Society of America
7910 Woodmont Avenue, Suite 300
Bethesda, MD 20814-3015
800-3AUTISM (800-328-8476),
x-150; 301-657-0881
http://www.autism-society.org

National Autism Hotline/Autism
Services Center
605 Ninth Street
Pritchard Building
PO Box 507
Huntington, WV 25710-0507
304-525-8014

BIRTH DEFECTS
Birth Defect Research for Children
930 Woodcock Road, Suite 225
Orlando, FL 32803
800-313-ABDC (800-313-2232);
407-245-7035
e-mail: abdc@birthdefects.org
http://www.birthdefects.org

March of Dimes Birth Defects
Foundation
1275 Mamaroneck Avenue
White Plains, NY 10605
888-663-4637; 914-428-7100
e-mail: resources@modimes.org
http://www.modimes.org

National Foundation for Jewish
Genetic Diseases
250 Park Avenue, Suite 1000
New York, NY 10177
212-371-1031

BLOOD DISORDERS
The Leukemia & Lymphoma
Society
1311 Mamaroneck Avenue
White Plains, NY 10605
800-955-4572
http://www.leukemia-
lymphoma.org

Sickle Cell Disease Association of
America
200 Corporate Pointe, Suite 495
Culver City, CA 90230-8727
800-421-8453; 310-216-6363
http://www.SickleCellDisease.org

National Hemophilia Foundation
116 West 32nd Street, 11th floor
New York, NY 10001
800-424-2634; 212-328-3700
http://www.infonhf.org/

CEREBRAL PALSY
United Cerebral Palsy
Associations, Inc.
1660 L Street NW, Suite 700
Washington, DC 20036
800-872-5827; 202-776-0406;
202-973-7197 (TTY)
e-mail: ucpnatl@ucpa.org
http://www.ucpa.org

CHILD ABUSE AND NEGLECT
American Humane Association,
Children's Division
63 Inverness Drive East
Englewood, CO 80112-5117
800-227-4645; 303-792-9900
http://www.americanhumane.org

Kempe Children's Center
1825 Marion Street
Denver, CO 80218
303-864-5252
http://www.kempecenter.org

CLEFT PALATE
American Cleft Palate-Craniofacial
Association and Cleft Palate
Foundation
104 South Estes Drive, Suite 204
Chapel Hill, NC 27514
800-24-CLEFT (800-242-5338);
919-933-9044
e-mail: cleftline@aol.com
http://www.cleft.com

Wide Smiles
PO Box 5153
Stockton, CA 95205-0153
209-942-2812
e-mail: info@widesmiles.org
http://www.widesmiles.org

CYSTIC FIBROSIS
Cystic Fibrosis Foundation
6931 Arlington Road
Bethesda, MD 20814
800-344-4823; 301-951-4422
http://www.cff.org

DEAFNESS AND HEARING DISORDERS

Alexander Graham Bell Association
for the Deaf and Hard of Hearing
3417 Volta Place NW
Washington, DC 20007-2778
800-432-7543; 202-337-5220;
202-337-5221 (TTY)
e-mail: agbell2@aol.com
http://www.agbell.org

American Association of the Deaf-
Blind
814 Thayer Avenue, Suite 302
Silver Spring, MD 20910
800-735-2258; 301-588-6545
(TTY)

American Society for Deaf Children
PO Box 3355
Gettysburg, PA 17325
800-942-ASDC (800-942-2732);
717-334-7922 (Voice/TTY)
e-mail: asdc1@aol.com
http://www.deafchildren.org

Deafness Research Foundation
575 Fifth Avenue, 11th floor
New York, NY 10017
800-535-3323; 212-599-0027
(Voice/TDD)
http://drf.org

Helen Keller National Center for
Deaf-Blind Youths and Adults
111 Middle Neck Road
Sands Point, NY 11050
800-255-0411; 516-944-8900;
516-944-8637 (TTY)
http://www.helenkeller.org

National Association of the Deaf
814 Thayer Avenue
Silver Spring, MD 20910
301-587-1788; 301-587-1789
(TTY)
http://www.nad.org

National Deaf Education Network
and Clearinghouse
Gallaudet University
800 Florida Avenue NE
Washington, DC 20002
For information about children,
202-651-5051 or 202-651-5052
(TTY)
For information about adults, 202-
651-5050 or 202-651-5068 (TTY)
e-mail: Clearinghouse.Infotogo
@gallaudet.edu
http://ClercCenter.gallaudet.edu/
InfoToGo/index.html

DOWN'S SYNDROME
Association for Children with
Down's Syndrome
2616 Martin Avenue
Bellmore, NY 11710-3196
516-221-4700
http://www.acds.org

National Down's Syndrome
Congress
7000 Peachtree-Dunwoody Road
NE
Lake Ridge 400 Office Park
Building 5, Suite 100
Atlanta, GA 30328
800-232-6372; 770-604-9500
e-mail: ndsccenter@aol.com
http://www.ndsccenter.org

National Down's Syndrome Society
666 Broadway
New York, NY 10012
800-221-4602 (helpline);
212-460-9330
http://www.ndss.org

Parent Assistance Committee on
Down's Syndrome
208 Lafayette Avenue
Peekskill, NY 10566
914-739-4085

EATING DISORDERS
The American Anorexia Bulimia
Association, Inc.
165 West 46th Street, Suite 1108
New York, NY 10036
212-575-6200
http://www.aabainc.org

Overeaters Anonymous
6075 Zenith Court NE
Rio Rancho, NM 87124
505-891-2664
http://www.OvereatersAnonymous.
org

EPILEPSY
Epilepsy Foundation of America
4351 Garden City Drive
Landover, MD 20785
800-332-1000; 301-459-3700
http://www.efa.org

FOOD ALLERGIES
The Food Allergy & Anaphylaxis
Network (FAAN), www.faan.org

HIV/AIDS
Elisabeth Glaser Pediatric AIDS
Foundation, www.pedaids.org

AIDS Action Council
1875 Connecticut Avenue NW,
#700
Washington, DC 20009
202-986-1300

AIDS National Interfaith Network
1400 Eye Street NW, Room 1220
Washington, DC 20005
202-543-1202

The American Foundation for AIDS Research
120 Wall Street, 13th floor
New York, NY 10005-3902
212-806-1600
http://www.amfar.org

CDC National AIDS/HIV Hotline,
800-342-AIDS (800-342-2437);
800-243-7889 (TTY);
800-344-7432
(Spanish)

IMMUNIZATIONS
The National Vaccine Injury
Compensation Program (VICP),
http://www.hrsa.gov/osp/vicp
State-by-State Requirements,
http://www.cdc.gov/od/nvpo/law
.htm

JUVENILE ARTHRITIS
Arthritis Foundation
1330 West Peachtree Street
Atlanta, GA 30309
800-283-7800; 404-872-7100
http://www.arthritis.org

JUVENILE DIABETES
Juvenile Diabetes Foundation
International
120 Wall Street
New York, NY 10005
800-533-2873; 212-785-9500
e-mail: info@jdf.org
http://www.jdf.org

American Diabetes Association
1701 North Beauregard Street
Alexandria, VA 22311
800-DIABETES (800-342-2383)
http://www.diabetes.org

LEARNING DISABILITIES
Learning Disabilities Association
4156 Library Road
Pittsburgh, PA 15234-1349
412-341-1515
e-mail: ldanatl@usaor.net
http://www.ldanatl.org

National Center for Learning
Disabilities
381 Park Ave South, Suite 1401
New York, NY 10016
888-575-7373; 212-545-7510
http://www.ncld.org

MEDICALERT JEWELRY
MedicAlert Foundation
International
2323 Colorado Avenue
Turlock, CA 95382-2018
800-432-5378
http://www.medicalert.org

MUSCULAR DYSTROPHY
Muscular Dystrophy Association
National Headquarters
3300 East Sunrise Drive
Tucson, AZ 85718
800-572-1717
http://www.mdausa.org

NUTRITION
American Dietetic Association
216 West Jackson Boulevard
Chicago, IL 60606-6995
800-366-1655 (hotline);
800-877-1600;
312-899-0040
e-mail: infocenter@eatright.org
http://www.eatright.org

PSORIASIS
National Psoriasis Foundation
6600 SW 92nd Avenue, Suite 300
Portland, OR 97223
503-244-7404
e-mail: getinfo@npfusa.org
http://www.psoriasis.org

REYE'S SYNDROME
National Reye's Syndrome
Foundation
PO Box 829
Bryan, OH 43506-0829
800-233-7393; 419-636-2679
e-mail: reyessyn@mail.bright.net
http://www.bright.net/~reyessyn

SPECIAL NEEDS
Federation for Children with Special
Needs
1135 Tremont Street, Suite 420
Boston, MA 02120
800-331-0688 (in MA);
617-236-7210
e-mail: fcsninfo@fcsn.org
http://www.fcsn.org

Amend (Aiding a Mother
Experiencing Neonatal Death)
4324 Berrywick Terrace
St. Louis, MO 63128
314-487-7582; 203-746-6518

National Easter Seal Society
230 West Monroe Street, Suite
1800
Chicago, IL 60606
800-221-6827; 312-726-6200;
312-726-4258 (TDD)
e-mail: info@easter-seals.org
http://www.easter-seals.org

**The Children's Brain Tumor
Foundation**
274 Madison Avenue, Suite 1301
New York, NY 10016
212-448-9494
http://www.childrensneuronet.org

Pediatric Brain Tumor Hotline
University of Chicago
5841 South Maryland Avenue,
Room J331
Chicago, IL 60637-1470
800-824-0040; 773-834-3000

SPINA BIFIDA
Spina Bifida Association of America
4590 MacArthur Boulevard NW,
Suite 250
Washington, DC 20007-4226
800-621-3141; 202-944-3285
e-mail: sbaa@sbaa.org
http://www.sbaa.org

**SUDDEN INFANT DEATH
SYNDROME**
**National Sudden Infant Death
Syndrome Resource Center**
2070 Chain Bridge Road, Suite 450
Vienna, VA 22182
703-821-8955
e-mail: sids@circsol.com
http://www.circsol.com/SIDS

SIDS Network
PO Box 520
Ledyard, CT 06339
e-mail: sidsnet@sids-network.org
http://sids-network.org

**Sudden Infant Death Syndrome
(SIDS) Alliance**
1314 Bedford Avenue, Suite 210
Baltimore, MD 21208
800-221-SIDS (800-221-7437);
410-653-8226
e-mail: sidshq@charm.net
http://www.sidsalliance.org

TINNITUS
American Tinnitus Association
PO Box 5
Portland, OR 97207-0005
800-634-8978
e-mail: tinnitus@ata.org
http://www.ata.org

TRAVEL HEALTH

Immunization Alert

PO Box 406

93 Timber Drive

Storrs, CT 06268

800-584-1999

International SOS Assistance

8 Neshaminy Interplex, Suite 207

Trevose, PA 19053-6956

800-523-8661; 215-245-4707

e-mail: info@travelcare.com

http://www.internationalsos.com

Travelers Hotline

Centers for Disease Control and

Prevention

National Center for Infectious

Diseases

877-FYI-TRIP (877-394-8747);

888-232-3299

http://www.cdc.gov/travel

GENERAL HEALTH AND

INFORMATION

The American Medical Association

515 North State Street

Chicago, IL 60610

312-464-5000

http://www.ama-assn.org

The Centers for Disease Control

and Prevention (CDC)

1600 Clifton Road NE

Atlanta, GA 30333

800-311-3435; 404-639-3534;

404-639-3311

http://www.cdc.gov

National Institutes of Health

9000 Rockville Pike

Bethesda, MD 20892

301-496-4000

http://www.nih.gov

U.S. Department of Health and

Human Services

200 Independence Avenue SW

Washington, DC 20201

877-696-6775; 202-619-0257

http://www.os.dhhs.gov

U.S. Food and Drug Administration

Office of Consumer Affairs Inquiry

Information Line

HF1-40

Rockville, MD 20857

888-INFO-FDA (888-463-6332)

http://www.fda.gov

Index

About the Author

Lisa M. Chavis, R.Ph., is a practicing pharmacist and author of *Ask Your Pharmacist: A Leading Pharmacist Answers Your Most Frequently Asked Health Questions* (St. Martin's Press, 2001). Chavis is a leading expert in her field, between the feedback she receives from thousands of pharmacy customers, as well as her personal experience with numerous health care products. She is often called upon for product recommendations and health advice by patients, the pharmaceutical industry, and media.

Chavis is known as "The Drug Lady" from a dear customer who always asked for her by that name. He said that his doctor didn't have the time and the books he read didn't explain things in terms he could understand. Chavis has written pharmacy-related editorial content for almost a decade, including an "Ask the Expert" women's natural health forum for ThirdAge.com, consumer buying guides for wellness-focused Internet sites, and clinical pharmacy information for the popular online pharmacy Drugstore.com. Her fun and friendly style of delivering clear, understandable health information has won readers all over the world.

As an advocate for clear, understandable patient information, Chavis realizes that the pharmacist's duty is much greater than simply putting a label on a prescription. Advice about prescriptions, over-the-counter medicines, or drug interactions can mean the difference between a patient getting better or worse. She believes the pharmacist's role in the care of patients is comparable to that of the physician, because both are advocates for the patient's care and well-being, helping to direct them to the best solutions in a never-ending sea of products and therapies.

Chavis is active in the American Pharmacists Association (APhA), where she serves on the Policy Committee and in the Media Contact Group, where she has had the opportunity to speak to the media about the importance of quality patient counseling and appropriate drug information. She has appeared on the "CNN Weekend House Call," and her expertise has been noted in *Forbes, Business Week, Fitness, Ladies Home Journal,* the *Washington Post,* as well as other media outlets.

Chavis is on the Editorial Advisory Board of *Pharmacy Today,* a news-magazine for the pharmacy profession. She is also a frequent contributor and reviewer for the *Journal of the American Pharmaceutical Society* on the subject of over-the-counter medicines. She is well-respected by her peers in the pharmaceutical community and was voted Pharmacist of the Year in 2002 by *Drug Topics,* a top pharmacy trade magazine.

Presently, Chavis is a pharmacist in the Tampa Bay area of Florida, where she has ample opportunity to dispense valuable advice on proper use of sunscreen and sun care products.